BLOOD AND MEMORY

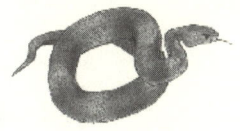

Robert Benson

Texas Review Press
Huntsville, Texas

Copyright © 2006 by Robert Benson
All rights reserved
Printed in the United States of America

FIRST EDITION, 2006
Requests for permission to reproduce material from this work should be sent to:

    Permissions
    Texas Review Press
    Box 2146
    Sam Houston State University
    Huntsville, TX 77341-2146

ACKNOWLEDGMENTS

I wish to thank Professor Rita S. Kipp, Dean of the College of Arts and Sciences at The University of the South, for her generous financial support. I am grateful to my old friend John V. Glass, Jr., for the original drawings of snakes and to Susan Blettel at The University of the South for the cover design.

Some of these essays have been previously published. "Rising to the Light," "Balancing Acts," "Charactered by Memory," and the poem "Grandfather" all appeared in the *Sewanee Review*. "Contours of Home" and "Tough Guys" were published in *Shenandoah*. "Out a Little from the Land" was published in *Southwest Review*.

This book would not exist without the particular help of two people. George Core, editor of the *Sewanee Review*, has for more than twenty-five years encouraged me to write, corrected my blunders, and lighted fires under me as necessary. I am grateful for his wise counsel and friendship. To my dear wife Ruth I owe more than I have words for. She is my first and best reader and critic and my reason for writing anything.

Library of Congress Cataloging-in-Publication Data

Benson, Robert, 1941-
  Blood and memory / Robert Benson.-- 1st ed.
    p. cm.
  ISBN-13: 978-1-881515-90-6 (hardcover : alk. paper)
  ISBN-10: 1-881515-90-7 (hardcover : alk. paper)
  ISBN-13: 978-1-881515-91-3 (pbk. : alk. paper)
  ISBN-10: 1-881515-91-5 (pbk. : alk. paper) 1. Benson, Robert, 1941- 2. Benson, Robert, 1941---Childhood and youth. 3. New Orleans (La.)--Biography. 4. College teachers--Louisiana--New Orleans--Biography. 5. Fathers and sons--Louisiana--New Orleans. 6. Heart--Diseases--Patients--Louisiana--Biography. I. Title.
  CT275.B5624A3 2006
  976.3'35063092--dc22

                                                               2006000839

BLOOD AND MEMORY

For
Robert and Andrew and Larry

In memory of
Lawrence and Powell

More than that, we rejoice in our sufferings, knowing that suffering produces endurance, and endurance produces character, and character produces hope.
—*Romans 5: 3-4*

. . . times saved by memory from the abyss into which most minutes, hours, days fall, unremembered and lost. —Ward S. Allen

Table of Contents

Introduction — viii

"Grandfather" — 1

1. Rising to the Light — 4

2. Balancing Acts -- 22

3. Out a Little from the Land — 46

4. Tough Guys — 62

5. Charactered by Memory — 86

"A Beastly Tear" — 107

6. Contours of Home — 108

7. The Heart's Sorrow — 128

8. Epilogue — 151

Introduction

If you've had a couple of drinks, you should not train the dog or discipline the children. When my sons were boys, I was enthusiastic about duck hunting and bought and tried to train my first Labrador retriever, a willful and wandering bitch we named Jessie. She was a beautiful yellow pup, playful and sweet-breathed, just the kind of dog the children could enjoy. I was ignorant and inflexible, and I wanted a dog whose retrieving deeds would impress others and reflect well on me. I've never been much of a wingshooter, but if I had an impressive enough dog, maybe no one would notice. The yellow Labrador was not yet the companion of every mail-order catalogue model, nor had it yet become the canine image of the American dream of financial success, but even then the power of image drew me. Ruth and I have had a lot of dogs in our forty years of marriage, and for most of those years my interest in them was tainted by vanity. Having a dog around may have helped domesticate us, especially me, although we consciously resisted referring to or treating our dogs as children, but it also fed my self-absorption. Jessie was not the first to be baffled by my eccentric expectations, my insistent mastery. I expected loyalty and obedience as elements of natural order. I saw no need to earn either. If a parent insists on obedience "because I'm your father," there must be a context of love and authority to make that more than mere intimidation and an admission of failure.

Vanity is a kind of heart trouble. It is a hard vice to outgrow and is less and less appealing as we age. It's easy to forgive the boy of thirteen who wants to dress like a movie tough guy and smoke cigarettes. Only when older will he recognize how silly and soft he really looked with his shirt collar turned up and a cigarette hanging from his lower lip. It's harder to be patient with the same vice in a forty-year-old who grows a moustache and affects a wide-brimmed felt hat and tall boots laced outside his pants legs because he wants to look like the duck hunters in faded old sepia-toned photographs. In a beautiful essay on horses, Thomas McGuane writes:

> Hunting on horseback, following bird dogs through an oak forest, which I have done with indescribable pleasure and a hint of self-satisfaction perhaps at the very picture I imagined myself conveying, seems a coherent activity in which man and horse and dogs, birds and forest coalesce into something of duration.

There's much to admire about that sentence, but one of its most remarkable features is the honest admission of the self-satisfaction that comes from imagining how one looks. Vanity asserts its claims even in an activity like hunting on horseback, which requires alert concentration and readiness.

I had the hat. Jessie was simply another part of the outfit. That she never sank her teeth into me testifies to her loyalty and patience. That I gave her reason to bite is beyond question, and she found more sophisticated ways to repay me. Being a bookish sort, I assumed that the way to get started training a dog was to read a book. I read Richard Wolters and Bill Tarrant and James Lamb Free. I read everything then available, and if there had been videos, I would have watched them. In the evenings before supper, I'd splash a little bourbon in a glass and take Jessie out for a training session. In the beginning it was easy. Labs do enjoy fetching dummies, and she was eager to please in those days, quickly learning *sit, stay* (if it wasn't too long), and *come*. I used a check-cord during basic training, and I actually thought having an impressive obedient retriever was going to be a snap. When Jessie was still under a year old, she was pretty good at marking the dummy's fall, and she was easily making double marked retrieves. Evenings, when she'd done especially well, I would go back inside and have a bit more bourbon and get Ruth and our sons to come out and watch her and applaud my way with dogs. With an audience, however, my patience became short, and my commands sounded not just forceful, but angry. An edge came into my voice, and if Jessie were a little slow to duplicate the retrieve she had done well without spectators, I would jerk her collar. She was, of course, baffled by my transformation, and her performance deteriorated accordingly, but the deterioration only increased my frustration. I could feel anger like a weight behind my sternum, and the only relief came as I raised my voice and treated her roughly. My heart may have been telling me something even then.

What I knew for certain was that something was on the line when my family was watching, something that I was desperate to retain by any means: my authority, the illusion of control. And the means that made sense to me were anger and force. I saw nothing peculiar in that. The boys were puzzled, though they had occasionally experienced my sudden tempers. Their sympathy was with the dog, and they found reasons to drift back inside. Ruth sanely and sweetly encouraged me to be patient and followed them. And whisky only makes vanity more sensitive, anger more grim. Conventional wisdom has it that a couple of drinks help one to relax, but, as often as not, those same drinks have the opposite effect and can make mere inconvenience or the exuberance of children or the stubbornness of an untrained pup seem like a deliberate affront. I had seen it all before and should have known better, but red whisky and yellow dogs went together, the liquor as essential to the images in my head as tall boots and double-barreled shotguns.

What I saw as wilful disobedience in the field or in the yard was nothing of the kind, but I did not understand. My anger swelled suddenly, and if I could catch her in some act of defiance, I screamed my disapproval and hit her. Before Jessie I had never understood Shakespeare's fiftieth sonnet in which the speaker lashes out at the horse carrying him from his beloved:

> The bloody spur cannot provoke him on
> That sometimes anger thrusts into his hide;
> Which heavily he answers with a groan.

The spur is bloody when brought into the poem since anger, frustration, and loss require a target. The horse can only groan. Reflecting on my shameful ignorance and cruelty, I am astonished that Jessie did as well as she did. My anger ruined many duck hunts. The beauty of dawn on a fiercely cold morning, wings whistling in the dark, the company of friends sharing a steaming thermos of coffee—all the pleasures that draw us to duck blinds—were of no consequence as I ground my teeth. The fate of Dante's wrathful mired in the marsh of Styx for being "sullen in the sweet air gladdened by the sun" is terrifying. In thirteen years of living with Jessie, I managed to learn something about not taking myself too seriously. I became a bit less concerned with the approval of companions and strangers, a bit less firmly attached to my vision of myself as some latter-day Natty Bumppo. I apologized to Jessie for my impatience and ill-temper, and she pretended not to remember. Our dogs since Jessie have had an easier time of it, and they owe her a lot. I shouldn't have been surprised when the doctor said I needed a triple by-pass and then a pacemaker. Jessie knew all along I had a heart problem.

Until my father's death, I lived in a world whose features and limits he defined. My adolescent rebellions were simple matters of bad behavior, the selfish excesses of the young, for it never occurred to me to raise fundamental questions. Even after I married and had children, I tended to accept an undiscovered world that had simply been delivered to me intact without ever wondering if it were real or fanciful or otherwise distorted. I am still puzzled and slightly embarrassed by conversations with contemporaries who struggled with the received wisdom of their upbringing, who fought their fathers out of some urgent necessity to discover themselves. In many ways my father was a strange man, and we had some angry confrontations in the course of our lives, but though I challenged him on particular matters, I did not doubt that his assumptions about the world were correct. I did not think much about the ways in which events of his own life had shaped his views. He was my father, and for many years that was enough.

The recollections in these essays centered on my father and his influence on my life and the life of my family began to take shape shortly after his death in 1981. In the days following his funeral, my brother Larry recalled the sadness and violence of our father's childhood, and I realized that I had not thought about the worst of these things since I first heard them as a small boy. Andrew Lytle's *A Wake for the Living* begins with this sentence: "Now that I have come to live in the sense of eternity, I can tell my girls who they are." As I have considered what my father saw and suffered, I have tried to imagine his childhood, his haunted memory, to make myself see. I wish I had done it while he was still alive.

In 1914, when he was a boy of eight, he witnessed his older brother's death in a bloody accident, and soon after that he was sent away to military school. Four years after his brother was killed, he was bitten by a rattlesnake. From that time and for the rest of his life, he carried a weight of sadness, fear, and rejection that I was insensitive to until he died. Since he said little openly about his feelings concerning these things, I had no reason to consider them, and as a child I thought my father behaved the way other fathers did. When I noticed differences, I ignored them. My mother, of course, knew more about his experiences and feelings than I did, and that knowledge, I now realize, is part of her role in my life, which has not always been dominated by the masculine world, as these remarks may seem to indicate. She tried hard to teach me to read what she called "the storm signals." When my father died, I was forty and my own life as a husband and the father of two sons had been profoundly affected by his more or less hidden past. Nearly fifteen years later I began writing about my father and about my boyhood in an attempt to understand him and myself. "Rising to the Light" was the first of these recollections, and in it I set down as clearly as I could my sense of the horror of my father's early life. As I began to tell his story, I came to understand the depth of his lifelong suffering and to catch glimpses of his capacity for love, his yearning for healing.

My father is not directly present in each of the memories brought together here, but my own behavior is linked throughout to his example. His stern insistence on order, his sudden anger, and his emotional reserve deeply marked my character as a boy and a young man, as did his generosity of spirit and profound loneliness, his certainty that all earthly joys are fleeting. His presence in my life is the tissue that connects these autobiographical sketches and helps to explain my own response to mortal matters. The undiscovered world I had accepted and inhabited for so long was largely constructed from his experience of deep pain and the awful weight of responsibility never entirely discharged. In the *Confessions* St. Augustine writes this about memory: "The power of memory is great, O Lord. It is awe-inspiring in its profound and incalculable complexity. Yet it is my mind: it is myself." Although there is much I still do not understand, in writing about my father and some of my own experiences before and after his death I have discovered order and coherence in surprising events.

BLOOD AND MEMORY

GRANDFATHER

> It did not even alter its course, not fleeing, not even running, just moving with that winged and effortless ease with which deer move . . . .
> "Oleh, Chief," Sam said. "Grandfather."
> (William Faulkner, "The Old People")

I

Heart-shot, he sprang out of the rifle noise
As if alive, arching through the gray light,
Clearing the stream in one uncoiling leap,
And fell heavily, stranger to clumsiness,
Surprised as a fallen dancer, graceless.

He ran slower then, and horizontal
Bright horns worked the deep red earth
In a passion more desperate than love.
Wild eyes fixed on the trees beyond,
A fevered child's dark eyes afraid of rest.

II

As boys we learned the smell of death
Exhaled in grandfather's last dry kiss,
A smell sharp and old as predator's breath
Caught in thin gauze, a damp flag fluttering
Over his wounded throat and going slack.

That sweet tarnished smell hung on forever
In the canvas coat you've worn twenty years
To this small cabin built of cypress logs
He cut and skidded through the swamp alone,
Where hunters cough and snore like the dead.
And bone-gray dawns still brighten into scent:
Old mattress, swamp, and rutting buck and blood,
All keen reminders of his death and ours.
Grandfather's laughter drove the night away.
I hear him yet in your rich voice and laugh,
And know why now we stay up late:
Back in dark bunks that smell coils, rank and chill,
Patient, unblinking as a rattlesnake.

III

Unsteady, wounded by success, we come
Unnerved at being so ignored, so alive,
Shuffling schoolboys afraid to dance or speak
To girls whose quick bright eyes see everything,
Heart-sore and clumsy in the dying light.

The buck's wild eye darkens and grows dull
As supple legs draw up with slow intent,
And their last uncoiling tears earth and leaves,
Carrying him in the gathering dark
Forever beyond the range of rifles.

Embarrassed we look elsewhere, finally
Certain that neither victory nor cold
Makes us tremble before his antlered head.

1. RISING TO THE LIGHT

My father believed that the only good snakes were dead, and he had better reasons than most people for this conviction. In the summer of 1918, he was twelve years old. In his yard near a sluggish creek, he was pushing his baby sister in the swing that hung from the lowest branch of an enormous live oak. Of course he was barefooted, and each time he pushed he stepped out of the way, usually stepping out from the tree. The swing rose higher and his sister squealed happily and threw her head back to watch clouds, branches, and bright sky flying past. The boy who would be my father enjoyed her delight and worked up a sweat trying to get the swing higher. The effort absorbed him and in his own yard he grew incautious. As he danced out of the way of the rushing swing and swiped at his sister's auburn hair as it floated by, he brought his bare foot down among the roots of the oak squarely onto a rattlesnake, and the small pit viper put both fangs into his right foot just above his big toe. It took Grandmother several minutes to get from the frightened child a reasonable idea of what had happened, and because she had another child, she thought first to kill the snake. In the time it took to dispatch the snake, my father's foot had turned a grayish green to the ankle, and his toes began to round as if filling with water.

Grandfather did not cut but he did suck. He put his mouth to the darkening wound, again and again sucking blood and venom from his son's swollen right foot. The doctor from town would not see the boy for twenty-four hours. That night, trying to do the right thing, his parents wrapped the foot in hot towels to "draw the poison," and the skin split across the top of the swollen foot. The bite of pit vipers hurts like a kidney stone, and rattlesnake venom is especially painful. The boy's fever rose, and he tossed on his bed and shook his head, knotting and unknotting his fingers, biting his lip and his forearm, not crying much. In August heat, he shook with cold and asked for more cover, but as a patchwork comforter was laid across him he screamed with fear. He experienced what he referred to for the rest of his life as "the horrors." Each patch on the comforter was a writhing snake coiling and striking repeatedly. He could not explain his horrors then, and the quilt stayed on. Blood poisoning, loving but primitive treatment, and the restlessness of recovering twelve-year-olds added up to nearly four months of recuperation. He remembered for the rest of his life the hemotoxic venom burning in his flesh, but another event in what should have been his childhood gave snakes their full mythic and symbolic weight.

Some things you never get over. Some terrible memories enter the blood and become almost genetic, touching even the lives of people who have no recollection of them. My father was never reluctant to speak of his snakebite. With little prompting he would re-create the incident in language plain and grim. But there was something worse that he would not talk about, not even with my mother, to whom he told nearly everything. It is an unruly and disproportionate matter, one of life's dark extravagances which can bring clarity to the lesser confusion of all our stories.

    When he was eight, my father saw his older brother beheaded in a mine shaft in Colorado. I recently came across an old photograph of a handsome sandy-haired boy, tie slightly askew, double-breasted jacket buttoned. The boy is smiling a pleasant, slightly smart-aleck smile. The picture seems well composed and complete, but the right side has been neatly torn away. On the back in my father's hand is this inscription: "Geo. Powell Benson—Lawrence's older brother—killed in Colorado 6/30/14." When we were children, without drama or self-conscious fanfare of any kind, my father told my brother and me the story that contained few more details than the writing on the picture, told us once as if it were part of his obligation to the truth and never spoke of it again. The telling couldn't have taken five minutes, and all that I remember is Powell was decapitated and parents never recover from the death of a child. My brother may have been old enough to hear such a tale, and he has told me other things about the accident and its aftermath that I do not remember. My childish imagination could find nothing to hold, and the telling sank within me like a polished steel weight. But in my fifty-third year that picture of Powell coupled with the fears fathers have about their children brought it all back, and I have tried to visualize the grim details of what my father suffered.

    The train ride from Louisiana in 1914 must have taken a week, but the boys had never been on a train, and they didn't care how long it took. Everything was fun. Grandmother was glad to see the country, relieved to have convinced my grandfather that the boys needed such a trip, that travel, as her mother had always said, was important to a child's education. She believed in expanding horizons literally. My grandfather grumbled some about their going and stayed home. Two days out of Kansas City, when the adventure had begun to flatten with the country, they caught sight of the Rockies. My father and Powell were thrilled, and Grandmother forgot the fatigue and the dust. She was convinced again that it was all worth it. The high country was delightful and exciting. Elevated vistas are not common in south Louisiana, nor is cool weather in June.

In Idaho Springs, they rode a buckboard to their hotel. On the way, Powell, who was eleven or twelve, saw a sign advertising tours of a played-out gold mine. "Can we please go, Mother? We might find some gold. It wouldn't take long. Please." My father took his cue from his brother. "Can we? Please? It's a real gold mine! Let's go see. Please." Grandmother was sweet-natured and liked to indulge the boys, and they knew if they kept begging that she would agree. Two days later Grandmother finally said yes. They would go to the mine on the next to last day of the trip. The boys danced and whooped in the hotel lobby, and Powell frogged my father's arm.

The mine itself was not much of an attraction, but the idea of going down into the earth greatly appealed to the children. The shaft cut into solid rock was not neatly squared, but four huge timbers supported the shaft and provided a frame to which the elevator was attached. The vertical supports, banded and bolted to the dark rock, were squared at the top and every 50 or 60 feet down by horizontal beams. Between each set of horizontal timbers, the bare rock, cool and wet in some places, dry in others, came close enough to touch. The elevator itself was a heavy wooden platform with an angled iron railing around it at waist height. It was raised and lowered by an old steam generator that the boys could hear grinding and slapping even near the bottom of the shaft.

The day was brilliant and clear, and looking up as they descended, they could see the huge pulley wheel that moved the elevator and beyond that, blue sky, a vivid piece of the bright world they had left. The shaft itself was dimly lit by a string of bare light bulbs that hung straight down on one side. The opposite side was either totally dark or shadowed and vague. The boys could tell when the rock walls were almost against the sides of the elevator by the sound of the clanking cable and the pulleys. Once or twice on the way down the platform even touched the rock. On the dark side, the boys felt the fenders on the lower edge scrape by. They leaned over and tried to touch the cool rock. The elevator operator and tour guide was no more than seventeen, but he was growing a moustache and enjoyed his authority.

"Keep your hands off that rock," he said with worldly irritation. "This ain't the playground. Gold mine's no place for kids." He said "kids" with deliberate disdain. My father giggled at the young man's accent and poked Powell in the ribs. Powell grinned back, and both boys leaned out for the wall again, leaning this time farther than they'd intended because the uneven rock had opened slightly.

"You'd best look to your kids, lady. They's ways to get bad hurt down here."

"Lawrence, keep your hands down," Grandmother said. "Powell, you boys settle down." The close rock walls and the deepening gloom made her a little anxious. She looked at her shoes and wondered if she had done the right thing.

It didn't take long to see the mine, nor did it take long to see why it had been abandoned. The boys' notion of finding gold lying about on the ground vanished in the dull gray horizontal tunnel. The guide walked slightly ahead with a coal-oil lantern, and Grandmother brought up the rear with another. The guide recited a string of dates dealing with the discovery of gold in the area and the construction of several of the local mines. His recitation on the mining process was as boring to the children as repetition had made it to him. Grandmother feigned interest so that the young man would not be offended, and she tried to ask questions she thought the boys might like to ask. The guide did not like having his speech interrupted by questions. It was hard enough remembering it all anyway. The boys made faces behind the guide's back and said they wanted to go. The elevator ride had been fun.

Going up, Grandmother spoke to the guide, but for the edification of her family of the hopes and fears that had brought men to these dark places. My father said you couldn't pay him to work in a hole in the ground, no matter what, and he fixed his eyes on the growing patch of sky overhead. He and Powell reached out to see if they could touch the rock. The elevator operator had stopped paying any attention to them. The platform rose with surprising speed, and near the top, Powell leaned over the railing to see if he could still see the bottom. As he leaned out, the platform passed through one of the sets of horizontal supports near the top. The sudden appearance of the timbers startled him, and he pulled his head back for an instant, smiled at my father, and leaned out again. Just above those supports a rock shelf came nearly to the iron railing. Powell's head and neck were between the rock and the railing as my father turned to him, mocking the guide. "This ain't the playground." He was still forming the words when the platform lurched and his brother's body fell at Grandmother's feet. The elevator rocked back and forth, its cable groaning as the platform settled. There was blood on my father's high leather shoes. He tried to look away, but his eyes could not find the sky. The charged air was full of his mother's screams.

In the summer of 1914, my father was eight. He was bitten by the rattler four summers later, but the two events became in some ways a single horror for him. He could never talk about Powell's death, for his own childhood was over from that moment. Four years later his sense of the uncertainty of life in the world was confirmed, and snakes became for him the embodiment of evil, darkness, and the promise of pain and loss, "evocative," as Faulkner says, "of all knowledge and an old weariness and of pariah-hood and of death."

From early childhood, my brother and I enjoyed hunting and fishing, hiking and camping, and we occasionally encountered snakes without disastrous results. Our father encouraged our outdoor interests, taking us fishing, teaching us to shoot rifles and shotguns, and whenever we encountered snakes, he killed them all regardless of name or reputation. When we walked in the woods, we had to walk behind him, follow single-file in his footsteps. He was an enthusiastic fisherman most of his life, but he never forgot the danger that waited on the banks of blackwater bayous. We never saw him as reluctant to go fishing or to be in the woods, but he was minutely careful, and we sensed that even a simple fishing trip was an adventure, fraught with real peril. It was very exciting. He was uneasy though on family vacations. If we went to Biloxi or Gulf Shores, we were made fearfully conscious of the dangers of the undertow. Once in Tennessee, we went to Rock City, probably at my insistence. I was ten. I remember running to the edge of the scenic overlook where I was supposed to be able to see seven states. I was stung and puzzled by my father's sudden anger. Neither of us enjoyed the afternoon. Mother described herself as a deathwatch Mary because of her anxiety about her children's safety, but my father's sense of life's tragic potential was vivid, if unspoken, in painful and bloody memory.

My interest in snakes must have been a particularly heavy cross for him to bear. Early fascination he expected to pass, but as fascination deepened and began to take on the look of science, he must have felt haunted, must have wondered what he'd done to deserve such a strange child. By the time I was thirteen, I had determined to become a herpetologist. Friends with a fondness for amateur psychology suggested that my father's loathing of snakes actually caused my interest, that knowing and not fearing snakes was a way of asserting my adolescent independence, a more civilized and acceptable way than juvenile delinquency, with which I had only a slight brush. As a second son, they said, I reveled in the other side of my father's fear. However that may be, I was conscious only of the fact that herpetology offered me an opportunity to combine academic matters with love of the outdoors. I read every snake book I could get my hands on, my favorite being Raymond Ditmars's *Snakes of the World* (1931), which contained a gory and precise account of Marlin Perkins's reaction to being bitten by a gaboon viper. I learned the scientific names for all of the common southeastern snakes and for many of the exciting snakes from far away places: the king cobra, the bushmaster, the Australian tiger snake. Being able to see a garter snake and say *Thamnophis sirtalis* was great fun of what I took to be a very mature sort.

A friend of my brother's got a job one summer

working in the snake house in the Audubon Park Zoo, and I immediately volunteered to be his assistant—at no salary. That summer I spent nearly every day at the snake house. I helped clean exhibits, washing windows, replacing gravel and water in the smaller tanks. My position was never official though I acted as if it were, moving confidently and with studied disdain through squeamish crowds, going nonchalantly in and out of the door marked POISONOUS SNAKES. NO ADMITTANCE. EMPLOYEES ONLY. I am certain now that no one noticed, but the summer after my eighth-grade year I believed I ruled at least a portion of the world, and I remember being mystified that the girls I longed to date remained unimpressed. When school started again in September, I spent three or four afternoons a week at the zoo doing whatever needed doing, delighted for the chance to observe and enjoy the snakes.

Although the snake house was small, dim, and damp, we saw and cared for an interesting variety of snakes, including some snakes that were rare even in grander zoos. During nearly eighteen months of my devoted service, we received and displayed two African cobras, a large and ill-tempered western diamondback (*Crotalus atrox*), a Mexican moccasin, an anaconda, and two Russell's vipers. The diamondback never adjusted to captivity, and we were not able to keep him on display because he would not accept the presence of people, striking repeatedly at the glass at the front of his tank until his nose and lips bled freely. He refused to eat and for several months he was force fed. He struck the wire walls of the holding cages with such force that his fangs would occasionally get caught in the hardware cloth. We turned him over to one of the herpetologists at Tulane. The cobras, on the other hand, adjusted quickly to their circumstances. We received two adult African cobras from another zoo, and for a day or two in the holding cages they would "hood up" and hiss loudly when anyone walked by. But they soon ignored all human activity, and we opened the door to their cage casually to freshen their water or to drop in the rats upon which they fed. My recollection of the offhanded way with which I moved among dangerous snakes now makes me a little nervous. Youthful reflexes and some knowledge yield only an illusion of invulnerability. My world held no horrors to moderate my confidence.

The snake house also had a good collection of local snakes: canebrake and pigmy rattlesnakes, water moccasins and copperheads, king snakes, rat snakes, ribbon snakes, a mud snake, a hognosed snake, and an assortment of water snakes. In fact, my first nonpoisonous snakebite was from a large diamondback water snake. I was cleaning one of the walk-in exhibits. It was the job I liked best. I wore red-soled rubber boots with my jeans tucked down inside and brought in a garden hose with a trigger-controlled nozzle. Visitors were always impressed by seeing a person in a snake tank (a "pit" they liked to say), even if the snakes were nonpoisonous. I hosed out the enclosure and cleaned the glass front with a squeegee. The bigger the crowd, the more nonchalant I tried to be, reaching down to move knots of snakes out of the corners with my hands. All snakes have rows of recurved teeth for holding and swallowing prey, and the larger the snake, the larger the recurved teeth. Diamondback water snakes are not only large, but they are intractable and ornery. As I reached for the tail of one snake, another snake that I had ignored bit the back edge of my right hand. Because the snake's teeth are recurved, the best response is not to jerk your hand away, but to allow the snake time to free his teeth and pull back. The best response, however, takes a lot more self-control than I possessed. As soon as I felt the bite, I jerked my hand, dislodged several of the snake's teeth, and helped him make a rather spectacular if superficial wound. I was embarrassed to have been so careless in front of an audience and pleased to have been publicly wounded. "No ma'am, I'm fine. Thanks. It's part of the job. Really. I'll be fine." A week later at school, I pulled a perfect recurved tooth from my hand. It came out just like a splinter.

My activities in the zoo and as an aspiring herpetologist did not escape my father's notice, but he was generous and tried not to interfere. He had over the years built several cages to house the generations of hamsters that had once interested me, and he did not pay too much attention to the fact that these cages provided temporary housing for snakes, and he never saw the copperhead that escaped from one of these cages in our garage. I'm still not sure how it got out, but snakes are adept at improbable escapes. I never mentioned it. Now and then, in the arrogance of youthful knowledge, I presumed to instruct my father concerning his attitude toward snakes. One Saturday morning my mother woke me up saying, "Son, go see what kind of snake that is your father killed in the yard." I was angry before my feet hit the floor. Why couldn't they have called me before he killed it? Why should I get up now? It wouldn't be any deader in an hour or two. Pulling on my jeans, I walked into the back yard still rubbing the sleep from my eyes. My father had put the hoe away and was spraying the insects on the camellia bushes. "Where's the snake?" I asked. He gestured with the hose on the stirrup pump toward the roots of the magnolia tree. There I found a black racer cut into three sections. The tail was lifting and turning slowly. "It's a blacksnake, *Coluber constrictor constrictor*," I announced. My father paid no attention. He didn't need to have his adversary named. "Dad, it's just a blacksnake. They eat mice. It's not poisonous. They're good to have around."

"No live snake's good to have around." He smiled, glanced at the three pieces of snake, and went back to spraying the flowers.

I said "shit" under my breath and started back to the house.

"Son, when I walked out past the magnolia, that snake came toward me," he offered in explanation to dignify my position.

I knew too much to let it pass. "Blacksnakes are aggressive like that sometimes. But he couldn't have hurt you. His pupils are round. He's nonpoisonous. You didn't have to kill him." My tone was smug and instructional.

"Who do you think you're talking to?" he said. Herpetology was no longer the subject. "I don't intend to get close enough to check the shape of his pupils. Anything I can't see from the end of the hoe, I don't need to see. And I don't need a lecture from you. Is that clear?" When I muttered "yessir," he turned deliberately away and walked back to the flowers.

Occasionally I rescued nonpoisonous snakes from his wrath. In fact I thought he almost admired a green snake, *Opheodrys aestivus*, he watched me catch, but when I mentioned it to him later he just laughed. "They're all ugly as sin, every kind there is." Nothing I said or did ever saved a venomous one. The truth is I didn't try often. Canebrake rattlesnakes, *Crotalus horridus atricaudatus*, are not numerous over much of their range, and although I had seen others catch them, I had never collected one. My father had asked my brother and me to help him clear brush from the banks of a muddy creek that ran behind the house. It was August, and even though we had started before six in the morning, we had sweated through our shirts and jeans by seven.

My brother said, "Let's sit a minute after I knock this privet down."

"You got it," I responded. I never had to be told twice to stop working.

As Larry swung his brush hook into the tangle of privet, we immediately heard a rattler buzz. We probed gingerly at the sound and discovered a twenty-four-inch canebrake. When we prodded the snake, he assumed an impressive posture, raising the front third of his length in a striking loop and trying in vain to retreat against a wall of cut brush. He rattled continuously. My father had been twenty or thirty feet down the creek bank when the rattling started. He was moving closer as I started up to the house for my potato rake and a pillowcase.

"Watch him. I'll be right back," I called to Larry.

As I moved past my father, he caught my left arm in his left hand and spun me toward him. "No," he said.

"Daddy, I've never caught a rattlesnake. This one's a perfect size for the collection. We've got a medium tank that's empty now anyway." I pulled my arm free, and I started to the house. I took a step and saw him pick up my brush hook and move closer to the snake.

"Please, Dad," I said with more anger than supplication.

He looked from the snake to me. I took one step in his direction, and he raised his left hand with his index finger pointing up at my face. His own face was flushed. His lips did not move much.

"Not another word." Each word was louder than the one before.

I stopped. The first swing took the snake six inches behind the head and cut him neatly in two. The rattling continued until there were not enough connected muscles left to move the tail.

My father's feelings toward snakes never changed. As he grew older, he was outdoors less, and encounters with snakes were unlikely. My enthusiasms moderated some, and time made both of us more good-humored about matters herpetological. In June after my freshman year in college, we went bank fishing on Bayou Lacombe on the north shore of Lake Pontchartrain, and I watched him kill a large cottonmouth that swam into the roots of a cypress tree near our stringer of bream. He went to the task with purpose and warmth, losing his cap in the process. As he flung the dead snake from the end of a heavy stick, he looked over as if he expected me to intercede belatedly on the snake's behalf.

"Protecting our fish?" I asked. We both laughed.

Coral snakes (*Micrurus fulvius fulvius*) are the rarest of Louisiana's poisonous snakes, or at least the most rarely encountered. They are slender and brightly colored little snakes which are sometimes mistaken for harmless snakes by those Ditmars calls "misguided persons." In his *Field Book of North American Snakes* (1939), Ditmars describes the coral snake as "a very dangerous snake from a combination of deceptiveness in appearance and actions and the high toxicity of its bite. . . . Of coral snakebites that the author has heard of, two out of three were fatal." The neurotoxic venom is, Ditmars writes, "drop for drop more lethal than that of a cobra." I had collected or observed nearly every species of native poisonous snake in my herpetological ramblings, but I had never seen a coral snake in the field. In fact, only one of the experts I knew had ever collected one.

I fished a lot the summer after my freshman year in college, and on several Saturdays my father went with me. One morning, however, when I proposed fishing, he declined.

"You go on," he said. "Your mother and I are

going to transplant a couple of those smaller camellia bushes, and I want to do it before it gets too hot."

"Do you need some help?" I asked without enthusiasm.

"No, thanks. Go fish. Just don't catch 'em all."

I was gone most of the day, but I have almost no recollection of fishing. When I pulled into the driveway around 4:30, Mother ran down from the porch to greet me. She was excited. I turned off the key and stepped out as she announced, "Your father's caught a coral snake!" And then, more modestly, "At least that's what we think it is. Come and see."

We walked around the house toward the garage. In the back yard my father was watering the bushes that he had moved while I fished. Near the door to the garage was a big glass jar with a piece of 2 x 6 lying across the top. In the bottom of the jar there was some leaf litter and a couple of pieces of moss. I knelt down to look closely.

"I figured if there wasn't enough air in there with that board on top, to hell with him," Daddy said as he turned off the hose and walked over.

There was a coral snake in the jar, and for several minutes all I could do was look. Then, "Where was it? Who saw it first? What did you say? How on earth did you get it in the jar?" The questions rushed out. My father smiled.

"I saw it when I got ready to dig out that second bush. It was just there, inside hoe range too. I was ready to smack him, but your mother stopped me. She had just seen the snake and said, 'Lawrence, wait. Don't kill it. I think it might be a coral snake. They're rare. And very poisonous Bob says.' You can imagine how impressed I was.

"Anyhow, your mother made me keep the damned thing at bay while she went looking for one of your books. It took her forever, but then she appeared with a picture and stood there looking first at the book then at the snake. 'Yes,' she concluded, 'it's a coral snake all right. I think we should try to catch it.' I don't recall agreeing to anything, but she found that jar in the garage."

"Your father was magnificent," Mother offered. "He looked like he'd been catching coral snakes all his life. I put the jar down and your father lifted him on the shovel and dropped him in and then shoveled that moss and stuff in for him."

"For him nothing," my father said. "On him sounds better. I thought it might kill him." He smiled and touched my shoulder.

While I listened to this remarkable narration, I lifted the jar and turned it around to look at the small, bright snake. My father never looked at the jar, showed absolutely no interest in its contents. Throughout the account of this adventure that he never could have imagined, his tone was cheerful and matter-of-fact. But he only looked at me, occasionally at Mother when she offered some detail or correction, and every now and then he looked off as if he were listening to something faint and far away that only he could hear. That evening he looked tired and old, but he was relaxed and went to bed earlier than usual and slept soundly.

It's been more than seventy years since Powell was killed and my father was bitten, and I have tried to find a place in memories that are not mine. I have tried to imagine the horror of an elevator ride out of a gold mine I have never seen. I have tried to look at snakes as he saw them all his life without trying: still bright with a child's fear and bewildering pain. Some things are clear now, but much of what I remember puzzles me. I also know that I have said and done much that puzzles my sons.

Daddy caught the coral snake when he was a year or so younger than I am now. My children have played with and learned a lot about snakes, and my wife has been a patient if not an enthusiastic home zookeeper for thirty years, but when I passed fifty I grew uneasy about a number of things. Age brings caution, and I am more or less constantly aware of what might at any moment be lost. I have never worried much about my sons being harmed by poisonous snakes. I worry because they live in a world more dangerous than the Honey Island Swamp ever was, a landscape of burnt-out gold mines, tawdry and dark places that promise what they cannot pay. I am grateful when I can deal with threats directly. Recently an old friend and I were walking with our children on his land along the Alabama River. We walked through the open river-swamp woods in single-file, at my suggestion. Jack led the way, his son and daughter behind him followed by my sons and me. I have always walked in the woods paying as much attention to the ground as to anything else, an old habit of my father's solidified by my years of snake collecting. We saw a few deer, flushed a wild turkey hen from her nest, and watched pileated woodpeckers and a variety of songbirds. We were nearly back to the truck when I looked ahead and noticed that Jack and his daughter had just stepped over and his son was about to step on a thirty-inch rattlesnake. I lunged by my two sons and grabbed Jack's ten-year-old and pulled him back.

"Snake," I said loudly.

"Where?" Jack asked.

When I pointed to the snake coiled in the leaves, Jack said, "Damn. I stepped right over him. So did Liddell." He shuddered. "Good eyes."

The snake had not moved since I first saw it. It neither rattled nor attempted to escape. I shot it once with a small .38 and watched as it knotted and rattled. I told myself that I was protecting the children.

I have an old black-and-white photograph of my father steering an outboard motor on a cypress skiff down Bayou Lacombe. He is laughing and looks young and confident. At forty-seven he could enjoy some of the things he had missed as a boy and a younger man. For a time after the accident in Colorado, his mother, nearly mad with grief and guilt, held séances in the dining room to bring Powell back. Night after night my father heard his parents pleading with the dead, terrified that his brother's mangled body would move through the house. Having come out of the gold mine alive, he also felt guilt and saw reproach in his mother's eyes. The year before he was snakebit he was sent away to military school. The grace and courage with which he lived into his seventies are apparent in his laughter and most vivid for me in his improbable encounter with the coral snake, a reckless act of love unimaginable until performed. When he died two months before his seventy-fifth birthday, he smiled like a housebound boy given permission to go and play.

2. BALANCING ACTS

Some men of my father's generation wore neckties and jackets when they hunted and fished, although the world was becoming casual. Whatever he wore, my father was not casual. Most of my childhood he worked six days a week. Many weeks he made six and a half by going to his office after church on Sunday afternoon. He was a lawyer and a man whose formal bearing preserved old civilities and kept others, including members of his family, on their mettle and at a distance. His own childhood was marked by pain and the bloody accidental death of his older brother, and he had learned well to guard his emotions. Like most of his generation, he managed without psychoanalysis, counseling, or therapy. He managed by ritual and custom, relying on traditions of manners and the military courtesy and order he had grown comfortable with at the Gulf Coast Military Academy in the years following his brother Powell's death. He managed with deep confidence in God's Providence. He bottled up a lot, living and working with a stiff upper lip. No one ever thought him frivolous. He slept, worked, and ate on a schedule, all business of daily living attended by forms of movement and speech carefully observed and habitual. In some ways, I suppose, he was not easy to live with, but the world of my childhood was stable and predictable largely because of the order my father imposed and insisted upon.

Sidney Champagne was a trapper who lived somewhere around Lake Salvador. No one could have dreamed a man less like my father, and yet he was the only man I ever heard call my father by his last name without putting "Mister" in front of it. Sidney usually came to visit in the fall. He would appear on our porch and knock, and when he saw my father coming toward the screen door, he would say, "Hey, Banson. Les go hunt dem docks." My father always smiled because it was Sidney and said, "Wait till I get my gun." Both men laughed. They had known each other since before I was born. They had hunted big ducks on Lake Salvador and Bayou Couba and had fished for redfish and specks, not as sport and guide, although it would have been easy to assume that, but as friends. I learned these things from Sidney. He had also paddled my father far out into the marsh so that he could take depositions from trappers wintering in remote tarpaper shacks. Sidney had inherited his pirogue, carved by his father with axe and adz from a huge cypress log, and Sidney handled it with either pole or paddle with the easy efficiency and precision that come from years of daily use.

As a younger man Sidney had made a good living in the marsh, trapping muskrat, mink, otter, and coon, doing a little market shrimping and crabbing, and selling crawfish in season to a few local restaurants. When an exploding nutria population made trapping unprofitable, Sidney refused to leave the marsh for the steady income of oil-company salaries even though many of his neighbors insisted that was the only sensible option left. Jerry Autement, Sidney's closest neighbor, tried hard.

"Hell, Sidney, damn nutria everywhere. Who you kiddin'? You can't do dis n'more, no. You and yo ol' lady gon' starve. You can't make a livin' off dem nutrias. Tings change, man. You look out for yoself."

But Sidney would not leave. He claimed he was too old to learn new work; only trapping and fishing made sense. My father said Sidney was too independent and ornery to work for anybody but himself. He met Sidney not long after he started practicing law. The marsh was Sidney's home, and he knew not only where the trappers' cabins were; he knew where most of them ran their lines. Most he could find in less than a day even when the weather was bad. Sidney and my father must have hit it off from the start. Long after he quit going into the marsh to interview trappers or to hunt or fish, he and Sidney kept in touch.

Sidney came by the house whenever he was in New Orleans. In the fall, if the ducks were down, he would propose a hunt. My father rarely did anything out of the way, but now and then he would accept Sidney's invitation and make plans to go. When was always a problem. Sidney wasn't much for schedules that the marsh didn't set, and my father's routine did not allow for spontaneity. The hunts they planned usually ended up being postponed once or twice and then canceled. After a visit to the house, Sidney would call a few days later if cold weather had brought ducks in ahead of it and say, "OK, Banson, les go." I could hear that much even though my father held the phone. Occasionally Sidney would begin their conversation with duck calling. He used his natural voice to call ducks, never a manufactured call; and if you looked away, you could not have said with certainty that you were hearing a man, not a duck. My father would begin to shake his head slowly as he listened. Sidney would talk about the weather and huge flights of ducks. My father would smile and say with what I took to be genuine regret, "Sidney, this is a bad week. I've got things on my desk I just can't quit on, and I'll be in court most of next week." Sidney said something that made my father laugh. Then, "Good luck, Sidney. Don't kill all of them, and don't freeze to death out there. It'll be in the twenties Wednesday. Thanks for calling."

I loved listening to their conversations on our front porch. Even as a child I remember thinking what an unlikely pair they were. They were roughly the same size, my father only slightly taller and thinner. Sidney looked at least fifteen years older than my father, for his life in the marsh had weathered and stained his face. His hair and stubble were gray. I remember him always in a brown wool jacket frayed and patched on the lapels and sleeves, a wool shirt, and brown canvas pants held up by narrow suspenders. Sidney reminded me a little of the movie actor Gilbert Roland whose role as a Cajun shrimper in *Thunder Bay* had greatly impressed a boy eager to grow up to be a trapper or a charter-boat captain.

On the porch after supper, my father would have unbuttoned his vest, but his tie would have been still in place. His starched white shirt seemed to provide its own soft light in the gathering dark. Both men smoked. Their talk was all of Sidney's world—the marsh, how many and what kinds of ducks Sidney had been seeing, how the trapping was going, how many nutria, how few muskrat or mink. Only when Sidney came did I hear such talk, but I knew that it was genuine and that it described a world I was longing to know. I loved Sidney for what he did, and I loved and envied him because he knew my father in a way I did not. It surprised me to realize how much my father knew about the life of the marsh and about the struggles of trappers and fishermen. He even seemed familiar with the details of setting a line of leg-hold traps.

It was hard for me to believe that my father had not always worn a tie, that he had grown up not in the city but in the rural South around the time of the first war. In the years marked by his brother's death and his own painful encounter with a rattlesnake, he had hunted and fished and gone barefoot, had milked cows and plucked chickens, had caught lightning bugs and gigged frogs, had run a trapline to make a little money. All that seemed unimaginable when I studied the dignified and austere figure at the head of our dinner table. Except for Sidney's occasional visits, however, my father rarely spoke of these things. If I asked him a specific question, he usually brushed it aside more or less gently as if my question had distracted him from something important. Later I realized that he had deliberately put that world behind him as if it were part of that childishness he had to put away as he had put away the old bolt-action .22 and the 16-gauge side-by-side that had belonged to his father. That he never gave it up completely is plain in the fact that he did not sell those guns, and he never gave up Sidney. I am grateful that he didn't.

When I was eleven or twelve, Sidney took me duck hunting for the first time. My father had arranged a hunt with Sidney for my brother, Larry, a few years before, and now it was my turn. It was as if my father knew that fathers should take sons duck hunting, but he was busy and not very interested in hunting anyway. I think he also knew that his tragic view might have cast a pall over the trip. Loading guns and inexperienced children in and out of duck blinds and pirogues is not something he could have accomplished with equanimity. Besides, Sidney was an expert, and I'm sure my father thought that would make for a better experience all around. At the time, I couldn't have imagined better.

Because he had no desire to spend the night in the hunting camp on Bayou Couba between Lake Cataouatche and Lake Salvador, my father and I got up around 1 a.m. to drive to Seller's Canal and take a motor launch several miles to the south. Sidney would be waiting for us at the camp. I slept in the car and woke as we crunched over oyster shells in a small parking lot. It was still black dark. Just off Highway 90 at the head of Seller's Canal there was a small grocery store where trappers bought supplies and where many of them left their hides. Three walls of the frame building were covered with stretched hides pulled tight over wire drying frames. The store was not open at two in the morning, but there was a light on, and I saw people moving around inside. A man stepped up out of the dark behind us and flipped a cigarette into the canal.

"Mr. Banson?" His voice sounded like Sidney's, but much younger. "We ready right over here. Dis all your tings?" He took the gun slip and the canvas bag with shotgun shells from my father and walked toward an elevated plank walkway.

"That's everything," my father said and slammed the trunk. I must have just been standing there watching my breath in the cold, still as much asleep as awake, because he then said to me, "You're not going to shoot any ducks in this parking lot, son. Come on."

I had never been in a strange place in the predawn darkness, and walking out on the planks after my father unnerved me. The boards sprang with my father's weight just enough to throw my steps off balance a bit, and I came close to falling. Being sleepy didn't help. I could not see anything below me except the tops of the water hyacinth, and in the faint light from the store

I caught a glimpse of black water and slick mud. Even the cold air smelled of dead fish and drying hides, wood smoke and coffee from the little store, and around it all the smell of the marsh itself, heavy and old, almost palpable in the dark.

Seller's Canal at the Highway 90 bridge resembles a waterway through a jungle. Even in January the woods look impenetrable from the canal. The canal starts on the southern edge of the great bottomland hardwood swamp that is part of the Mississippi and Atchafalaya River bottoms, and as the heavy crew boat headed toward Bayou Verret and Lake Cataouatche, it ploughed deep into black water. From inside the warm cabin, I watched the boat's impressive wake wash against willows and cypress knees and vanish into the timber. As we neared Lake Cataouatche, however, I could tell even in the dark that the horizon had opened. The night was clear, and I could see the great arc of the sky filled with stars. We had left the river swamp woods and were moving through the enormous and trackless marsh that extends clear to the mouth of Bayou Lafourche and the Gulf of Mexico. The boat's deep wake now seemed to lift the expanses of grass and rushes into rolling waves that moved into what looked like solid ground. After daylight I could see islands of live oaks that Sidney called cheniers. Except for those bits of high ground, the world was flat and brown to the horizon.

Sidney was waiting at the camp, standing out by the dock in the cold dark, smoking and listening to mallards on the water nearby. Inside the camp was too warm and the air smelled musty, a combination of mildewed mattress and stale whiskey, and in the light of a single kerosene lamp, unshaven men only half awake cursed and laughed softly. Pieces of conversation continued from the night before mixed with obscene recommendations for waking the lazy and hungover. I heard no mention of ducks except for a voice from a dark corner declaring that he would only shoot the ducks who tried to climb into bed with him.

"And then she took out her glass eye" produced general laughter. Someone noticed my father as he stepped into the light to get coffee.

"Hey, Larry. You didn't come down last night. You could have lost money like Chap did or feel like dogshit like I do. What are you—antisocial?"

"No, Paul, I just didn't want to expose this young man to trash so early in the day," my father said with a smile and lifted his chin in my direction.

Paul seemed only slightly embarrassed as he walked over and shook my hand. "Is this little Larry?"

"That's Bob. Sidney's going to show him how to kill a duck."

"Sidney? Is he around? I haven't seen that old coonass once this year. He slips in, he slips out. People claim to have hunted with him. I couldn't testify that he's still alive."

"You better watch that. He's alive and right outside. Son, come get this cup of coffee and grab a biscuit or two. Sidney doesn't like trash any better than I do. And besides, it stinks in here. Who died?"

"Oh my, a hunting camp that stinks. How odd," a voice spoke from under a quilt across the room. "Mr. Benson must be here. Watch your language, boys. The only man I know who comes down here expecting civilization."

"Go back to sleep, Charlie," my father said laughing. "Nobody should expect civilization who's likely to run into you."

Back outside the cold air made my eyes water, and I tried to warm my nose in the steam from my coffee.

Sidney was still down by the water. He didn't look as if he'd moved since we arrived.

"Dat's de same crowd, eh, Banson? Dey come to drink and play cards. Dey care nuttin' about dem docks. It's gon be good dis morning. Dem Franch dock cuttin' up all night."

He hadn't looked at us as we walked up. The eastern sky was just growing light, and Sidney was watching small flights of ducks pass into the less dark and disappear. A mallard hen hailed a passing flock from just a few yards away.

"Les go, boy. Where your gun and shells?"

My father handed the gun slip and shell bag to Sidney, who placed them carefully in the pirogue. "Banson, we'll bring you some dock this boy gon' shoot way before breakfast."

"You do just what Sidney tells you to, son. Sit still and don't rock the boat. It's too cold to go swimming, and pirogues aren't hard to tip. Good luck."

"Thas experience talkin', boy. But you don swim here any time," Sidney added seriously.

The pirogue rocked wildly as I stepped in and settled near the front, then steadied when Sidney stood and poled us out into the dark water. I looked around and saw my father walking back up the planks into the dim light of the camp house. I was cold, and in the dark I wished I had stayed with him. Sidney laid the pole alongside me, sat, and began to paddle. I could feel the pirogue surge with each quiet stroke, and there were ducks everywhere. Once or twice Sidney would stop paddling to listen as we drifted. When I looked back at him, he looked as if he weren't paying attention to anything. He picked at the duckweed stuck to the paddle. But then he would lift his arm and point. "Der he is." As the sky grew light, a twisting knot of teal overtook us from behind and flared over my head.

It didn't feel like we'd gone very far, but when we reached the blind, I looked around and saw open water and marsh grass in all directions. The blind was brushed out in cane and swamp myrtle and had a platform in it about three feet above the water, and Sidney stuck the pole into the mud as I stood and climbed out onto the rough boards. The sun was nearly up, and as I looked at the flat marsh, I thought I had never seen so much sky. There were wooden decoys in front of the blind, still and lifeless in the cold. I had heard Sidney talk to my father about live decoys, but they were no longer legal. A blackbird swayed on the tall grass and then flew.

"Which way is the camp house?" My fear of being thought timid always lost to my real timidity.

"Back over der." Sidney gestured with his head. "Now load dat gun and keep your head down. Dis clear sky dem docks see everting."

I was carrying the 16-gauge double that had belonged to my grandfather, the same gun that Larry had killed ducks with a few years earlier. What I didn't know then was that I am cross-dominant—right-handed and left-eyed—and that only by rare accident would I be able to hit a flying target. Other than that, the morning hunt was perfect. Sidney must have been puzzled and frustrated by my failure as a wing shot, but he never let on. His voice was as soft and steady on the last shot as it had been after the first.

"You gots to catch and pass dat bird and shoot where he gon' be, not where he's at." His blue eyes looked at me intently as he swung his left arm. "You done shot behind dat duck too. You ain't trying to scare him to death, no."

Sidney was also demonstrating the right way to kill a duck. He called to ducks flying high in the cold cloudless morning.

"Here dey come," he said around his hands and called again.

As far as I could judge, his calling was flawless. When Sidney raised his beat-up side-by-side twenty, ducks fell dead—two shots, two ducks. I didn't see him miss. I had never hit a flying target before, and I had no high hopes to be dashed, but watching Sidney cup his leathery hands at his mouth to call and seeing him swing without effort and drop ducks—one, two—filled me with admiration. Sidney was as much in his element as I was out of mine. He was as confident and relaxed as I was shooting baskets in my back yard. This was, in fact, his back yard, and if my self-conscious awkwardness was disappointing, he never showed it. Nor did habit make Sidney careless. He handled his gun, his boat, himself deliberately. Even mounting his gun suddenly at the appearance of unexpected ducks was accomplished without wasted motion. Spontaneous and liturgical could have described the same action. Hunting was fun, but it was also serious and potentially dangerous business. Sidney was the keeper of a rite, and in that he was like my father.

I did not go back to camp empty-handed. I was credited by Sidney with having killed a black duck and a canvasback, and I may have killed them. I have a picture my father took of me in front of the camp house on Bayou Couba holding those ducks. But recently I have wondered whether Sidney didn't simply shoot as I shot and let me claim the birds that fell. At this distance, it doesn't much matter. My memory holds Sidney, like a revered uncle or older brother, giving me a steady and privileged look at a world he loved, a world that was gone before I grew up.

When I was seventeen, I worked on a surveying crew based in Houma. We worked two-week pay periods, ten days in the marsh and four days off. In the marsh, we lived on the motor vessel *Captain Bob*, a 54-foot cabin cruiser that slept a crew of seven. The *Captain Bob* stayed anchored in the same spot for most of the summer. Every morning we loaded surveying instruments, brush hooks, and machetes onto the crew boat and headed into the marsh, one day in one direction, next day another. The workday was twelve hours, six to six. We took coffee and sandwiches with us. Larry had tailed chain with this crew in previous summers. His advice was simple: don't whine, and don't lose your sense of humor.

"The work's tougher than you expect, and everybody knows you're a city boy. If you act like you can't take it, they'll make your life miserable. Try everything and don't complain. You'll be all right. You do have to win their respect, but it's worth it. You'll be fine."

The regular members of the crew were men like Sidney except that they had left traditional ways of making a living in the marsh, opting for the regularity of survey work. Nutria had ruined the fur market, they believed, and the men on the crew complained that the shrimp and oysters were disappearing too. Nothing was as it used to be. They had families to feed. They still hunted and fished, did a little shrimping and even set traplines, but their lives and the lives of their children no longer depended on those things. Surveying in that watery world allowed them to use some of the skills they had learned trapping and hunting and kept them home, but some of the men in their thirties spoke wistfully about the lives of their fathers and cursed the nutria.

"Damn nutrias got tits on they backs. Belly fur al' tore up by de marsh, back fur wit tits. What good an animal like dat? Alligator bait, thas all." (In fact, the nutria's mammary glands are high enough on her sides so that the young can nurse while riding on their swimming mother's back.)

They suffered no illusions about the hardships their fathers and mothers had endured. Yet somehow, in those days, everything was better. Everybody told and retold stories of great trapping seasons, great duck hunts. Harry LeBlanc told me the same story all summer, about belly-crawling across a quarter mile of frozen marsh to ambush black ducks.

"Dat ice cut up my hand. I ain't had no glove," Harry said and flipped his long black hair out of his eyes. "Drag my gun backwards too. Fool Tony push his gun tru dat grass before him. Dat barrel ful of mud and shit whan he jump up to shoot. I was some cold dat day. Pants froze stiff on my leg."

In the summer, I learned a little about walking in the marsh on the floating mat of vegetation called the trembling prairie, the *flotant*, and I listened to unsentimentalized stories of a vanishing world, a world whose tangible traces I saw all through the marsh: abandoned winter camps of trappers, rotted pirogues disappearing slowly into the mud, the remains of a rough-planked dock, and occasionally a forgotten trap still staked, but long since sprung and rusting at the edge of a muddy slough. I picked up the first of these I found, and Parrison Landry said, "Jes trow it back. I tink thas probly one of ol' Baptiste traps. He bin dead tree, four years anyway."

The first morning I stepped off the crew boat onto what looked like solid ground, I sank through the floating mass up to my hips. The rest of the crew stood laughing, the tops of their shoes still dry.

"Hey, city boy," Landry said, "what you doin' down der?"

"You got to stay on top de marsh to walk," Harry LeBlanc added.

C. J., who was the surveyor, was laughing too hard to say anything, but he gave me a hand and pulled me up. When I put weight on it, my right foot sank back as far as my knee. C.J. still had me by the hand and pulled again.

"Shit, boy, you ain't come out here to swim, no. Hol' your feet so they don't take all your weight."

That advice makes no more sense to me now than it did the first time I heard it, and it was like the other bits of coaching I received: offered generously, but finally mysterious and untranslatable. I felt heavy and uncoordinated, the spastic member of a ballet troop. Harry LeBlanc tried to demonstrate how to walk the marsh by holding both hands out in front of his chest and moving them as if they were feet.

"Do like dis here," and he would move first his right hand and then his left. It looked to me like any attempt to describe any sort of walking. No help. Day after day, I fell through the marsh again and again. Most days I worked soaking wet, covered with stinking mud. Other members of the crew were only wet with sweat. During lunch break after a week or so, I told Parrison Landry I didn't think I'd ever get the hang of it. Parrison was the best marsh walker on the crew, and everyone acknowledged his superior skill. In particularly bad stretches of marsh where there was more water and less vegetation, Landry was the one who went ahead and found a route that most of the crew could follow. On a couple of those occasions everybody but Landry got wet. Those were the times I could only tag along by swimming and crawling. Landry got to laugh at everybody.

"Listen, Banson," Landry said, "you got to walk like a cat." He fixed me with his eyes and added without irony, "Slow and fass at the same time."

I think I could see it when Landry did it, but I

was not a quick study and never really got the hang of it. The most difficult walking involved crossing canals and sloughs that were being choked by grass floating in on lumps of dirt the crew called heads. These lumps had not yet rooted themselves to the body of the marsh. Stepping onto these heads was a little like stepping onto any kind of floating ball. As soon as you put your weight onto the lump of grass, it sank and shifted wildly. I watched Landry lead the crew across several of these sloughs. His balance and timing were perfect. Each step seemed calculated and deliberate, and yet he moved with such speed and grace that it also appeared as spontaneous as running. C.J. and Harry could frequently keep up with Landry, even carrying a range pole or transit and level, but sometimes when the head rolled under weight, one or the other of them would fall in always to Landry's delight.

"How you gonna teach dat boy to walk out here, clumsy as you are? He can' learn nuthin' watchin' dat. Dat boy grandmother can stay drier dan you."

In midsummer every year the crew was sent to Grand Isle at the lower end of Barataria Bay to work at the company's camp during the annual Grand Isle Tarpon Rodeo. Skilled hands like C.J. and Landry took boats out into the Gulf so that company guests could fish. The rest of us served as kitchen help and houseboys at the camp, making sure the guests had beer and whiskey, clean sheets and towels, fresh decks of cards and pretzels. We worked twenty-hour days for four days straight, being allowed to go to bed around ten and rousted at two in the morning to make sandwiches for the sports to take with them. The company used the Tarpon Rodeo to court men of authority and influence in the southern parishes and to reciprocate for various kindnesses: mayors, sheriffs, judges, police chiefs, state legislators. Many of the guests were men with names like Broussard and Guidry, Foret and Plaisance, whose fathers also had been trappers and fishermen. But these politicians and public servants prided themselves on seeing the future and recognizing the knock of opportunity. They didn't understand how their fathers could have been so blind. It was plain that the best living to be made from the marsh was not one that required you to get your feet wet or your hands dirty. The future was with the oil companies who would get what they wanted and whose gratitude was legendary. These men were both lazy and ambitious. Though they lived right next to folks like Landry and Harry LeBlanc, they held themselves aloof. As guests for the fishing tournament, they delighted in ordering men they had grown up with to fetch them a cold beer or a clean washcloth.

"Haarray, bring a fresh towel here. I like to rub something hard on my face in the morning," said a soft pink-faced man sitting on the edge of his bed, thin reddish hair falling into his eyes, his pale freckled shoulders lined by the sheets.

Raising his fist as he passed me with the towel, Harry LeBlanc whispered, "I rub dat sonofabitch face wid dis. I been knowing him since we was small."

In the evening when the boats were back in, Landry spoke with disgust about having to bait hooks for someone he had grown up fishing with.

"How a man forgets how to bait a hook? You got to forget everting to be a judge? Dey tell me what I got to forget, I tell dem, to hell wit being a judge."

Most of the complaining, as most of the patronizing, was habitual and formulaic. There were times, however, when it became serious and destructive. At the end of a day's fishing, one of the sports, a member of the state legislature, had dressed C.J. down in front of his wife and daughter. As I later learned, the legislator, a pharmacist from Cut Off, had hooked and lost a good sailfish, a fish he thought might have won a prize. After he had played the fish for a few minutes, it simply got away, hooked solid one moment, then slack line, the fish gone as if it had never been. No one was at fault, but the sport drank heavily all the way back to Grand Isle, and on the dock he was sullen and blamed C.J. for losing his fish, cursed and called him a dumb coonass who had no business taking anybody fishing. It took Landry and LeBlanc over an hour to persuade C.J. not to go after the lawmaker with a ball-peen hammer.

"Nobody talks to me that way in front of Lizbet and my little girl. If my ass need chewing out, fine, but you don't do my family dat way." His face was red, and the veins in his neck bulged. C.J. would not let Landry get hold of the hammer, and there was some pushing. I remember being afraid of what he might do. C.J. was strong as an ox, and I had never seen a man so determined to defend his honor.

"He ain't worth killin'," Landry assured him. "He sure as hell ain't worth goin' to jail for."

"I'm just gon' break that sonofabitch mouth so he can't talk dat trash no more."

Next morning the sober legislator was put on another boat and cautioned to stay out of C.J.'s way. He seemed shocked. "What's he pissed off about anyway? It was no big deal. That was a hell of a fish, you know."

Nothing came of it finally, but all the crew deeply resented those low-order politicos and hangers-on and main-chancers. Every summer men who were content to put in twelve-hour days in the marsh, who knew and loved that watery world and all its seasons and creatures went for four days to be the flunkies of men who held them in contempt, men whose only connection to the natural world was a paper one—deed and lease agreement—who would neither bait a hook nor set a trap, who disdained the very world they sought to profit from. They could have been from anywhere. Like convention goers, they came to Grand Isle forgetting manners and restraint. They drank too much and stayed up too late. Occasionally they puked in their beds, and Harry LeBlanc or I would be wakened to clean up the mess and change the sheets.

I haven't been in the marsh for forty years, but lately I have thought a lot about Sidney and Landry and the rest, about duck hunting and the Tarpon Rodeo at Grand Isle, about trying to walk the marsh. Even when I was a boy, roads and canals were beginning to provide the careless and incompetent easy access to a disappearing wilderness. The navigation and pipeline canals have also permitted saltwater to flow into freshwater marshes, and even places that look much as they did no longer support the same plants and animals. The Louisiana Department of Wildlife and Fisheries is trying to make trapping nutria economically attractive, and some eccentric optimists hope to add nutria to the list of popular Cajun foods. But there are still too many nutria and too few trappers. Trapping cannot compete with the petroleum industry's salaries and benefits, and the culture that sustained trappers is gone. The conflict now is a familiar environmental one. Bumper-sticker wars are fought with slogans such as SAVE OUR MARSH OR OIL FEEDS MY FAMILY, suggesting a complication neither side fully understands. So tourists can see what one looked like, an Acadian village has been built near Lafayette. In July of last year my wife Ruth and I were visiting in New Orleans, and I decided to go see what had become of Seller's Canal. My expectations were not that high, but my brother was not encouraging.

"Think, Bob. It's been, what, forty-five years since you went hunting with Pop and Sidney? There's probably a Wal-Mart parking lot on the beautiful banks of Seller's Canal."

I feared the worst, but Seller's Canal was still marked on a current map, and Ruth has always been a good sport about my fool's errands. Early one morning we crossed the Mississippi on the Huey P. Long Bridge and headed west on US 90. Subdivisions and strip malls had sprouted like toadstools around the Avondale Shipyards—an enormous operation and certainly that area's largest employer. We believed that Larry must have been right, but as we drove west, the land began to look slightly familiar and undeveloped. Closer to the parish line, the borrow pits on each side of the highway were choked with water hyacinth. Beyond the pits, a jungle of water oak and cypress formed a wall through which we caught occasional glimpses of standing water and expanses of marsh grass away from the road to the south.

Practically at the St. Charles Parish line, the road crossed a wide black-water canal completely covered in places by duckweed and hyacinth. On the left side of the road there was an old bar with a large tin garage or boat shed attached to the rear. The shell parking lot led down to a chancy-looking boat ramp, and down the canal we saw additional boat sheds listing at various angles toward the water. Aluminum jon boats were tied to pilings near the ramp, and around the sheds were a few larger wooden boats, some half sunk, all old and unrepaired. The air was thick with wasps and dragonflies, and the day was already heavy and hot, so unlike the cold days of duck season. It looked like the place I remembered. Except for the fact that the old store was now a bar, time appeared to have stopped around 1950.

As we pulled into the parking lot, a fisherman had just gotten his boat trailered and was turning out onto the highway. The heat had shut down the fishing early.

"Is this Seller's Canal?"

For an instant the man's face blanked as if I had spoken to him in Hungarian, and then he smiled slightly, privately, and said, "Yep."

I thanked him and parked in front of the bar. His response had been peculiar, something in the tone, and my confidence that we had found the right spot was shaken. Maybe he was just visiting and hadn't wanted to appear ignorant. The bar had no name; the sign in front said BOAT LAUNCH $2. The door was unlocked, but it was dark inside. We called out as we entered, but got no response. An old pool table with a broken cue lying on frayed velvet sat in the center of the room, and there were mounted fish and ducks on the walls. Behind the bar a bright sign said GEAUX TIGERS, and a lighted Budweiser clock turned slowly over the door to the men's room. We went back out into the glaring heat and walked around to the metal building. Inside, in a little clearing amidst trailers, small boats, and unidentifiable engine parts, hung a bare light bulb. Everything looked used up and abandoned. Even the partially assembled motors were dusty as if some mechanic had not come back from his lunch break twenty years ago.

An old man, who had apparently been down on the floor, stood up and began to rummage through the litter on the workbench. I was encouraged by his appearance. He wore cutoffs, stained deck shoes, and a thin white shirt. I could read the label on the pack of cigarettes in his front pocket. His face was weathered, and his stubbly beard was gray. I thought for a moment that he looked a little like Sidney.

"Good morning. Is this Seller's Canal?"

"What?" He looked startled to see anyone. I repeated my question.

"I don know. I'm not from here," he said in an accent that I couldn't identify.

"Dis here canal run to dat lake." He pointed over my shoulder. "Lake Cat, Cat, somethin."

"Lake Cataouatche?"

"Si. Das right, but I don know d'name of dis here." He gestured toward the canal.

"I duck hunted around here when I was a boy, but I haven't seen it in forty years. I'm going to take a few pictures if you don't mind." I held up my camera as evidence.

He had no interest in my connection to this place nor in my camera. I took several pictures, and we left. It looked right, but my confidence was shaken by the old man who didn't know where he was.

"Is this it?" Ruth asked when we were back in the car.

"I think so, but these people don't know and don't care. Let's drive a little farther toward Boutte and see if there's another possibility."

We continued driving west, and in another mile or so we crossed another canal that also looked right. A low, yellow brick building on the edge of the highway said, BARBARELLA'S LINGERIE. LIVE ENTERTAINMENT. Behind Barbarella's there was a small, well-kept frame house that was both residence and office for a boat rental business. The prices on the sign looked old: BOAT RENTAL - $3, PIROGUES - $2, BAIT - $1. The top of the sign read PIER II. A boy of four or five was relieving himself in the front yard. He was unembarrassed by our approach. Two nondescript dogs barked as we got out of the car, but neither one got up. I knocked on the screen door.

"Help you?" said a voice from inside the house.

"Is this Seller's Canal?"

A man who looked to be in his thirties walked out of the dark house onto the porch. His belly hung over his belt, and his expression was that of a man who has been asked a trick question and does not want to be taken in.

"Is this canal called Seller's Canal?" I pointed at the water so that there would be no confusion.

"I'm not from around here," he said. "We just call it PIER II." He pointed at the sign for clarity's sake.

I took some more pictures, feeling uneasy and slightly disoriented. An old black man was bank fishing beside his truck fifty or sixty yards down the canal. We walked in his direction. Clearly he was local. He looked like he had been doing this all his life. He was small. One leg was much shorter than the other, and his back was bent at an odd angle. I called out when we were still some distance from him to avoid startling him.

"Morning," he replied with a smile.

"Any luck?" I asked.

"Jus' got here." He had found a shady spot to sit, and there was a cooler on the bed of his truck parked a few feet away.

"Do you know if this is Seller's Canal?" I was beginning to feel foolish.

"O yeh," he said with conviction. "All dis here 'cella's—what his name . . . *Marcella.*"

We were not on the same wavelength, but I blundered on into this strange word-association game.

"Carlos Marcello?" I named the New Orleans crime figure, a man who was infamous when I was in high school and who had probably been dead for years.

"Yeh. He own all dis around here." He made a sweeping gesture.

Hell, for all I knew, he was telling the truth, but

it wasn't anything that helped me. I tried to get back to my subject.

"This must run down to Bayou Verret and into Lake Cataouatche."

"I don' know. I'm a bank fisherman," he said as if his preoccupation explained and precluded any interest beyond the shade he was sitting in. "Fishin's good here. Sometime bass, sometime sacalait. Dis morning I hope to catch me some perch."

We wished him luck and walked back to the car. Both places we had stopped reminded me in different ways of Seller's Canal on a cold, dark January morning long ago, but they were tended by people who weren't from here and didn't know where here was. I had never met so many people who seemed uncertain of where they lived and who were at the same time so unconcerned. Knowing where you are is a way of knowing who you are, and in the swamps and vast reaches of marsh beyond Seller's Canal, not knowing either of those things could get you killed.

Though everything was new to me, my first duck hunt was customary: movements, even language itself, shaped by traditions older than any of the living participants. And I was doing what my older brother had done. I was wearing his coat and using the shotgun he had used. I was riding in the same pirogue. That morning, if we were all near the end of something, I didn't know it, and my father and Sidney, who might have known, spoke only of ducks and the approaching dawn. As a small child, I had listened to my father and Sidney talking on our front porch, their voices naming places they both knew: Boutte and Bayou Lafourche, Grand Isle and Bayou des Allemands, Manchac and Barataria. I repeated those names to myself and found them spelled on maps, names rich with possibilities and suggestions of adventure. Older, I saw those places for myself, and on a cold morning in a duck blind beyond Seller's Canal, I felt I had claimed an inheritance.

I remember my father's voice warning me about how easy it is to turn over a pirogue, still remember watching him walk back toward the lighted camp house in the gray morning as his friend paddled me out into the marsh to a blind between Lakes Cataouatche and Salvador. While I was in high school, Sidney died poling his pirogue, running a line of traps not far from the duck camp. When his heart quit, he simply fell forward in the small boat. Jerry Autement knew where to look and found him just before dark stretched out in the pirogue built by his father's hands, laid out like some fierce old Saxon king, boat-buried, marsh birds keening.

3. OUT A LITTLE FROM THE LAND

I grew up in New Orleans in a house built at the start of the twentieth century not far from the Audubon Park Zoo. Summer after summer I fell asleep listening to lions, almost able to convince myself that I was in Africa. The heavy summer air was alive with insects that I never saw pictures of. They clicked occasionally on the warm sheets after Mother turned out the light. As I dozed off, I could hear the lions, coughing, growling, and grunting mostly, but now and then really roaring. The sounds, I expect, were magnified echoing off the walls of the lions' enclosure. J.A. Hunter writes that "A pride of lions on the hunt communicate with each other by deep grunts that have a strangely ventriloquial quality. It is almost impossible to tell where the noise comes from." Often I simply went to sleep. The big cats sounded far away, and the sound of my older brother's regular breathing from across the room was reassuring, but sometimes, in response to a lion that sounded close because the wind had changed, my heart raced and my body flushed and tingled, and I gripped the bed suddenly as if I were falling. At such times, I was convinced that the lions were loose, prowling the levee, bounding between the live oaks on St. Charles Avenue, finding my house. I longed for adventure as any boy does, but very early I also learned to be afraid.

My first adventures were imaginary, my imaginings formed by *The Boy's King Arthur* and *The Wind and the Willows*, by movie cowboys like Tom Mix and Lash Larue, by stories in *Field and Stream*, and by an assortment of cheaply printed and wildly inaccurate men's magazines I read in the barbershop, magazines with stories of attacking pythons and rogue snapping turtles. I remember very early thinking that if I owned a lever-action rifle and a gaff, everything would be all right; my problems would all be solved. The rifle and hook were tools of the life I imagined myself living, substantial and efficient instruments that conferred status and promised adventure. An awkward and clumsy child, I was an early subscriber to the modern notion that the right pieces of gear would transform me. Except for the fact that I had little money, I was an ad-man's dream consumer, but though I read *True* and *Argosy* at the barbershop and saved money to order a Wham-O slingshot and a blowgun advertised as capable of killing a wild boar, I remained a clunky and uncoordinated kid who secretly realized that being either a soldier of fortune or a charter-boat captain required experiences of danger and discomfort and plain boredom that I was not up to. That realization, however, never dimmed my fascination with the weighty tackle of lives I still admire and slightly envy.

My earliest real adventures were fully domestic affairs that took hearth and home to the wilds. The whole family watched me catch my first redfish just off Mobile Bay, and I caught my first fish on a fly under the approving eye of my mother. But those events paled before the real adventure of our first deep-sea fishing trip, trolling for Spanish mackerel out of Biloxi. The boat was a small, beat-up work boat called *Lucky Lady* with two primitive fighting chairs near the stern and without the sophisticated electronic equipment that today's fishermen regard as essential. I saw a compass and heard a radio. I have no idea how old the boat was, but all of the once varnished wood around the cabin had been painted bright blue, and where the paint was chipped you could see several coats beneath. The ceiling of the cabin was lined with enormous reels and short, thick rods rigged with streamers bigger than any fish I had ever caught. Across the stern in a rack that was both secure and accessible were the first two gaffs I had ever seen, one with a very short handle, the other with a wooden shaft nearly five feet long. They were beautiful. I knew what they were because I had seen pictures in magazines in the barbershop, but the captain would not let my older brother or me handle either one. The first time I asked, he just laughed. "Son, we don't need to be hooking one another. We'll use 'em if we get lucky."

The captain was a big man—fairly tall, I thought, and as big around as a barrel, but not fat. He was weathered. Every bit of exposed skin was deeply tanned, and his face was lined, like a dark version of my grandmother's face, I remember thinking. His hands were scarred and calloused, the well-used tools of a hard life. As we walked down the dock early in the morning, we saw him climb out of the engine well wiping his hands on an oily rag. He wore khaki trousers rolled halfway up his calves, and when he saw my mother, he ducked into the cabin and came back out buttoning a blue work shirt with no sleeves. He was courtly helping my mother aboard and loud and cheerful to Larry and me. His black eyes looked directly into mine. "You gonna be able to hold that big fish, boy?" he asked me. When I said, "Yessir," he laughed and turned to shake my father's hand. "Got two little fishermen there," he said, still grinning. "They sure want to be," my father responded.

Big as he was, the captain moved over his boat with graceful agility, never expending more energy than was required, but never hesitating to expend all that was necessary. Every move seemed familiar, habitual, from lifting a metal cooler full of ice off the dock onto the boat to selecting streamers and tying intricate knots. Ropes and fishing lines, which always seem to me to have a life of their own, went neatly where he wanted them.

Sport-fishing charters were still fairly new on the Mississippi Gulf Coast, and there was no mate on board. The captain did as much as he could but did not hesitate to ask my father for help. Larry and I did little things, but we were mostly in the way. My father released the bowlines as we backed slowly away from the dock, the boat's diesel engine growling and bubbling as small waves splashed over the exhaust. Two heavy trolling rods were stuck in rod holders on the fighting chairs. We traveled roughly southwest, out between Cat and Ship Islands. The hazy August morning brightened as we got farther from shore, and the waves were just big enough to feel like an adventure. I had never been on big water before, and when the islands disappeared behind us and the water turned clear and deep blue, I was afraid, but old enough to keep quiet about it. I looked at my family and wondered how we would manage shipwrecked on an island. My mind stuck momentarily on the image of my father unshaven in torn, shipwrecked clothes. I was about to ask him if he'd ever grown a beard, when the captain throttled back and said to Larry and me, "OK, boys, let's catch a fish."

As the boat crept forward at idle speed, the

captain lifted each rod and played out what seemed to him the right amount of line over the stern. One rod was rigged with a green and yellow streamer, the other a wide-bladed silver spoon. To the hook of each lure, the captain had added eight- or nine-inch strips of the dark flesh of some fish. My brother and I sat in the fighting chairs and received final instructions.

"Leave the rod in the holder between your legs," the captain said. "And raise and lower the rod tip slowly, like this. When you feel a fish, holler 'Fish on,' and I'll slow down while you reel him in. Nothin' to it. You fellas ready?"

We both said "yessir" at the same time, and the captain patted Larry's shoulder and left us. The boat changed direction and picked up a little speed. My father was standing near us, offering encouragement and advice, his tan cap pulled low over his eyes. He had white pants on and a long-sleeve, light-blue shirt buttoned at the cuffs and at the collar. He sunburned easily. I rarely saw my father without a coat and tie on, but I began to realize, as I watched him move about the boat and listened to his description of what the fish would feel like when it took, that he had done this before. It was as if he had a secret life of which I was catching my first glimpse. That was more exciting than not being able to see land. Mother was sitting forward in the shade. She smiled and waved as I looked to see where she was.

We trolled for what seemed a very long time without results, but then Larry caught a mackerel. He forgot to holler "Fish on," but I hollered for him, and the captain immediately slowed. As the exhaust grumbled and burbled through gentle swells, Larry reeled in his fish easily. Our luck improved from that point, and each of us caught several fish. The mackerel were small and no match for the heavy tackle we were using. After they hit the lures, they seemed to give up quickly, and we watched them sliding over the wake as we reeled. We caught a few dolphin. They seemed initially to fight harder than the mackerel, but they too were easy to reel in. Larry caught a small bluefish that really put up a fight. It dove deep when it felt the hook and actually put a creditable bend in the big rod. We were surprised at how small it turned out to be.

"I thought I had a monster," Larry said.

"Blues are scrappy." Daddy laughed.

"Wow," Larry said, mopping his forehead dramatically.

"That dolphin I caught was bigger," I insisted.

Mother and Daddy took turns in the fighting chairs, and each caught a fish or two. I was glad to take a rest, especially since it didn't look like there were any more bluefish around. It was fun to see Mother catch a fish. She laughed and was excited, even if it was just a mackerel.

Around two in the afternoon, we had all had enough, and Daddy told the captain that he thought it was time to head in. I was sunburned and tired; all that night I would feel the deck rising and falling under me. Daddy told Larry and me to reel in, and as we were reeling, the captain yelled, "Damn!" Then immediately to my mother, "Sorry, ma'am." He cut back to idle speed, pulled a rod off the ceiling, and stepped back near the stern. The rod was shorter and thicker than what we'd been fishing with, and it had only an enormous bare hook at the end of its wire leader.

"Boys, get those lines in the boat," he said as he took Larry's bluefish out of the cooler, ran his knife the length of the fish just under the backbone, and pushed the big hook through the fish's eyes. My father had spotted the shark by this time.

"That's quite a fish, captain. What'll he weigh?"

"Couple a hundred anyway," the captain said. "Maybe more. Let's find out."

He threw the bloody bluefish off to the side, and I watched as it landed a few feet in front of a hammerhead. The shark looked huge, its gray-green length moving lazily along just beneath the surface. At the bottom of swells, its dorsal fin came out of the water. The shark turned slightly as the bait hit the water. He wasn't more than thirty feet from the boat. He moved slowly past the bait as it sank, ignoring it.

"Damn. Sorry, ma'am," the captain said as he reeled in.

The shark didn't swim off. It swam in a slow circle as if it thought something more appealing might fall off the boat. I recall being at once delighted and afraid. To see such a large predator at ease in its natural element is to glimpse a great secret at the heart of things. Its presence reminds us of the frailty of our vessel, the vanity of our daily confidence. But it is also beautiful in its concentration, the economy of its movement, its sleek efficiency.

The captain threw the bluefish a second time. A second time the fish moved nonchalantly toward it. The bluefish was still very near the surface when I saw the shark's head lift out of the water, and the bluefish disappeared. The captain let the shark take line and calmly told my father to buckle on a rod holder. He still had not set the hook, and the shark was still moving lazily near the surface when the captain handed my father the rod.

"Hit him. Hard," he said as he moved back to the controls.

My father reeled very slowly until the line came taut, and then he suddenly raised his left hand, pushed down the butt of the rod with his right, and lifted the rod tip.

"Hit him again."

My father horsed back on the rod again.

"Again!" the captain shouted.

By the third time the shark had responded to the pressure, and the thick rod bucked in my father's hands and bent like a longbow. The fish had gone deep and was taking line fast. My father had pushed the butt of the rod into the holder at his waist and was bracing his left knee against the stern. I think he tried to laugh as he felt the strength of the fish, but he only blew out air as if someone were sitting on his chest.

For the next thirty minutes, my father fought the shark from one side of the boat to the other. The captain stayed at the controls, but his eyes never left my father. Occasionally he throttled forward just a little, and once as the fish made a long run, he reversed and the engine growled into its wake. Since my father had set the hook, we had not seen the fish. He fought as Larry's bluefish had fought, sounding constantly as if the depths would provide safety and release.

"He's coming up, I think," Daddy finally said in a strange voice.

The captain slowed the boat and spoke softly to Mother.

"Ma'am, if you'll come sit here and just steer for a minute. You don't need to do a thing—just keep us going straight at this speed. Don't you worry about doing anything. We're going be right busy back here, and it'll be a help if you just keep the boat headed out that way."

"He's coming up," my father said as if the words themselves were heavy and hard to handle.

After the captain put Mother behind the wheel, he opened a locked cabinet and lifted out a lever-action rifle, which I later learned was a .30-30. He worked the lever to chamber a round as he stepped back beside my father. Daddy's face was bright red beneath his cap, and his shirt was dark with sweat. I thought I saw his legs tremble as he adjusted his stance. His reeling looked awkward and jerky. Although he clearly knew what to do, this was not something my father did often. The rod was still bent, but the angle of line into the water was becoming less steep, and as my father continued to reel, the captain said, "There he is."

In the shadow of the boat, about twenty feet out, I could see the shark moving fast just beneath the surface. He didn't seem tired to me. The captain raised the rifle and fired three rounds at the head.

"Still a little deep," the captain said. "When he comes back around, raise your rod tip if you still can, and reel hard. One of those may have hit."

As I bent down to pick up one of the ejected cartridges, the captain moved to his left and knocked me down.

"Son, you've got to keep out the way now." He wasn't smiling, and no one was helping me up or even asking if I was OK. "You don't want to go overboard now." He looked down at me and grinned. I moved closer to Mother. She looked nervous steering the boat and only glanced at me.

As the shark came by the stern, my father pulled up hard on the rod, and as the great irregular head glided along at the surface, the captain fired twice, and pieces of shark popped into the air. My ears rang. The captain laid the rifle on the table in the cabin and grabbed the gaff hook with the long handle. The shark's tail was still swimming, but he could no longer resist the pull and direction of the heavy rod. I could see the wire leader abrading the front of his head.

My father said, "I'm about done in, captain. You'd best get that hook in him on the next pass."

"Don't quit on me now. Back up a step or two,

and bring him in close. When I hit him, move to the other side and keep tension on the line. Boys, you all go stand in there by your mother." He did not look at us, but we moved quickly, sensing that the tremendous fight was reaching a critical moment.

The captain leaned out over the gunwale and struck the gaff into the shark's far side just behind the gills.

"Move!" he shouted to my father as he heaved on the hook. The captain's face was red with strain, and the muscles in his back knotted beneath his shirt. He was only able to lift the hammerhead's front end level with the gunwale. Holding the gaff in one hand, he reached down and took hold of the nearest pectoral fin. He waited until the boat was in the trough between waves so that the next wave could help lift.

"Now," he said. "On my count, pull. One, two, three, pull!"

At first nothing seemed to happen, but then slowly the fish's great body slid up and fell onto the deck. The two bullets in the head had killed the fish, but its tail still beat loudly on the deck, and its mouth was opening and closing, gasping for water. The mouth seemed small to me, but the rows of teeth did not, and I could still see stringy bits of Larry's bluefish. When the thrashing stopped, the captain said I could touch the fish, and I ran my hand tentatively over the sandpaper skin. I had read that divers who hit sharks with their bare hands scraped themselves as if they had fallen on asphalt.

Back at the dock in the late afternoon, Daddy's fish drew a crowd. The shark was just under seven feet long and weighed right at three hundred pounds. People who did not know us at all shook my father's hand. Some of the other captains wanted to know exactly where we'd been, and strangers took pictures of my father and the fish. He was polite to everyone, but not happy with all the attention. I watched the captain closely as he cleaned up his boat. With the rifle put away and the gaff back in its rack, all signs of our adventure were gone, and in the years since I have even lost track of the pictures we took at the dock. But I could not have dreamed a better day, and the way the deck dropped under the weight of the fish and the feel of sharkskin have never left me.

Adventures in my parents' company, fishing or duck hunting, always lived up to my expectations. Their presence ensured order and safety, and even small mishaps I accepted as part and parcel of their plan. The passing of innocence surely has something to do with our increasing capacity to imagine or recall experiences that reality cannot match. Later, we are responsible for what order and safety we can manage, and that burden casts a long shadow. And much that we took for granted others would do, we must do unaided. My independent adventures have a tendency to go agley. In some ways, the real pleasure and clearest purpose of adventure for me is going home at the end.

In high school I read Hemingway. It was thrilling to discover that at last my teachers regarded as worthy the sorts of tales I had found so readable in the magazines of outdoor adventure I read in the barbershop. When I read *The Old Man and the Sea*, I could picture the great fish; the sharks seemed like my own memories, but I knew that alone in a small boat on open water I would be paralyzed by fear and uncertainty. Imitating the old man's adventure never entered my mind, but Bill Langland's taste for adventure required more actual participation than mine. It was Bill who first suggested that we try to catch a big fish—any big fish—on a hand line. He wanted something big enough to pull the boat. He was intent on duplicating the old man's competence and courage. A marlin was out of the question, but some of the crabmen on the north shore of Lake Pontchartrain told us that late in very dry summers sand sharks occasionally followed mullet schools into the lake. Another boy's uncle owned an eighteen-foot Lyman with a twenty-five horsepower Johnson outboard. Mark was sure his uncle would let us take the boat one Saturday. Lake Pontchartrain was not exotic, and the idea of real adventure close to home appealed to me.

Our preparations were, for three sixteen-year-old boys, pretty elaborate. We rigged two lines. Each consisted of one hundred feet of half-inch hemp to one end of which we tied six feet of fairly heavy chain. No shark was going to chew through that leader. To the chain we added an enormous hook. I do not remember the exact size, but our optimism was without bounds and showed in our hook selection. We tied several overhand knots in the end of the rope we would be holding. We would not wear gloves. For bait we caught mullet with our castnets. We took a six-pack of Jax into a white-hot July afternoon, launching Mark's uncle's boat at Irish Bayou. As we were about to pull away from the dock, Bill wondered out loud how we would keep the mullet off the bottom. We imagined that self-respecting sharks were not bottom feeders, and it had dawned on at least one of us that six feet of chain would not allow the bait to drift much. In a dockside trash can, we found a couple of one-gallon cans with screw-on tops and decided that they would serve us well enough as corks. Mark had a .22 semiautomatic rifle (I remembered that firearms were required for this work). And then there was the blood.

We all knew how useful chum could be in any sort

of fishing, and we had read enough to know that sharks are attracted to blood in the water and that they can follow a blood trail for amazing distances. The success of our trip depended upon blood, but quantities of blood are not easy to come by, and for a while we were stumped. There was in 1957 more than one abattoir in New Orleans, but when we called and asked if they would give us a bucket or two of blood, they hung up on us. I remember being puzzled by that abrupt reaction. Didn't they want to know why we wanted blood? One man said before he hung up, "You kids quit calling here." Was everybody going shark fishing? Bill's father worked at the Tulane Medical School, and he told us that dated whole blood donations could not be kept indefinitely even when refrigerated and that the medical school regularly disposed of old blood. He volunteered to bring us a few pints. We were thrilled. The idea had been proposed by a doctor, and we were not at all squeamish.

Coming out of Irish Bayou into the lake, we went more than halfway across and dropped the anchor about halfway between the highway and railroad bridges. We tied the oilcan floats just above the chains, baited our lines by hooking the mullet through both eyes, heaved the strange rig as far from the boat as possible, and watched as the wind drifted the oilcans away from us. We poured approximately four pints of old blood off the stern and cut up one or two mullet and pitched them over. And then we sat back, opened a beer, and waited. I cannot speak for Bill or Mark, but I did not expect anything to happen. I had never fished unaided by knowledgeable adults for anything more substantial than a bluegill, and I could not imagine this trip as anything more than an elaborate way to spend the day on the water and sneak a beer.

I first saw the oilcan go under about forty-five

minutes after we set it out. I had fished a lot with a cane pole and a cork, and I knew that sometimes the drag of the bait and a bit of wind can make your small cork look like a fish is taking your bait when it's not, and I think that was my first thought. My second thought was that that could not be true of a sealed one-gallon can. By the time both thoughts had flashed through my mind and before I could say anything, the can resurfaced.

"We just got a hell of a nibble," I said, pointing to the can bobbing calmly.

Mark and Bill looked and as the three of us watched, the can disappeared again. I grabbed the line and pulled hard, but I felt nothing on, and the can immediately reappeared. I pulled the line all the way to the boat to check the condition of the bait. There was not much tearing of the bait, but there were several punctures made by what looked like round teeth. It didn't look like shark work, but our minds were too full of shark to allow room for other possibilities. I threw the can, chain, and mullet back.

"Next time let him take it for a minute or so," Bill said. "That's got to be a hell of a fish. You know how hard it is to hold a can full of air under the water?"

Around ten minutes later, our cork again went under and stayed. We waited for what seemed hours but couldn't have been more than thirty or forty seconds, and Bill and I both hauled hard on the rope. For a moment we felt nothing, but the oilcan stayed under, and we began to take in line. I felt as if we had snagged something heavy but inanimate because there seemed to be no living resistance. A log, I thought, and when I first saw it, I still thought log. That an alligator gar can resemble a log in murky water will surprise no one who has ever seen one of these armored survivors. He was hooked, but offered no fight until he got close to the boat. By then it was too late. The stout rope held, and as he thrashed on the surface next to the boat, Mark emptied his rifle's magazine into the fish's head, and we unceremoniously dragged the creature aboard. The gar was roughly five feet long, and we estimated his weight at around sixty pounds, not nearly big enough to have pulled the boat even if he'd tried. A gar is not a candidate for a role in an heroic fish tale, and as we looked down at this sluggish throwback to the age of dinosaurs, the whole business seemed a waste.

Mark said, "My uncle's going to kill me. That damn thing's bleeding all over the boat. Throw it back."

"You're nuts," Bill said. "Back at the dock they'll take pictures of us. One of them might even make the papers."

Occasionally the local papers ran pictures of unusual catches from the lake, and ours would surely qualify. That would be a way to salvage our failed shark hunt. Having our picture in the paper might not make us heroes exactly, but it would be something.

"We're not going all the way back to Irish Bayou with that thing bleeding everywhere." Mark was firm about that.

"Fine," Bill said. "Let's cut a length of that rope."

I cut the hook and chain off one of the lines and then handed Bill about four feet of rope. He ran the rope through the gar's gills and out his mouth. The fish was still bleeding heavily as we lowered him over the side near the stern and tied the rope to a cleat. The boat was a mess, and Mark was worried about being killed by his uncle. He was out of patience with the whole business. Bill and I assured him that we'd help get everything cleaned up after we had our picture taken, and when he got the motor started, Mark headed for the boat ramp at full speed. As the heavy wooden boat got up on plane, the gar began to plane too, and as waves hit the fish, it began to flip up and down on the short rope. This was not *The Old Man and the Sea*. I hollered to Mark to slow down and pointed to the wildly bouncing gar, but just as he pulled back on the throttle, the gar's teeth or the back edge of his gill plate or both cut cleanly through the rope. The fish bounced off the next wave and sank like a stone. There one second, gone the next. We had no pictures, only a bloody boat and an odd assortment of empty containers: beer cans, hospital blood bottles, and two oilcan floats. The list looks more like part of an evidence inventory in a police investigation than the leftovers of a grand adventure. It hadn't been a bad afternoon, but in some ways that perhaps I should have been able to foresee, it was normative. At sixteen I couldn't see it, but expeditions that depend in part or entirely on my skills with ropes, knots, boats, guns, or hooks are doomed, not to the grand failures of Promethean struggle, but to low comic mediocrity.

I still hunt and fish, but I am not adventurous, nor am I much of a threat to wildlife. I'm still more likely to kill a coot than a canvasback. I would rather go out the back door and hunt rabbits in a familiar woodlot than go deep into vast river-bottom swamps, rather catch an occasional rainbow in my over-fished and heavily stocked home water than be dropped by floatplane alone near some remote and pristine Alaskan river. I have seen a wild bear, but I would not have abandoned watch and compass for the privilege. Undoubtedly I have missed much. I have heard lions and have always dreamed of Africa. But the safari that fires my imagination is itself domestic, lorries and bearers carrying more than creature comforts, bringing hearth, company, and all the blessings of home. The best of my real adventures are thick with images of my father, my brother, my sons, a few old friends, adventures that ended with a warm bath, my wife's kiss, and our familiar bed.

4. TOUGH GUYS

His name was Buddy Gianelli and he had a brown belt in karate. I don't know where Bill met him, but they had hit it off immediately, not just because he was a tough guy, but because he was interested in the same things we were: fishing and shooting, messing around in the woods and in boats, and he owned a Ruger single-six. Bill Langland and I lived in the same neighborhood and went through high school together. Buddy went to Jesuit, I believe, and I don't think I ever knew where he lived. He said that he had put a sailor in the hospital for making a pass at his girl, and we believed him. I saw the girl once, and she looked exotic and worldly. Buddy was a couple of years older than we were. He may have flunked fifth grade or started late or done something else. He seemed exotic too. His eyes were dark, and he slicked his black hair with aromatic tonic from the barbershop. He looked like what he was—like a Catholic from New Orleans.

Bill spent a good bit of time with Buddy in the spring of 1958, and one weekend the three of us went to the Gianellis' fishing camp in the Honey Island Swamp a few miles outside of Picayune, Mississippi. I was always a little uneasy around Buddy, but his invitation sounded a little like a challenge, so I couldn't say no. We planned to play cards and run a trotline in the swamp, checking it periodically through the night. Though I had no clear notion of what a trotline was, I thought it sounded like fun, an adventure of the sort I imagined constantly as a boy. We might even drink a little beer. Mother allowed me to drive her car, a Plymouth station wagon with push-button shifting and an impressive V-8 engine. Teenagers don't think much of station wagons, but the powerful engine made up for the lack of style.

We drove to Picayune on a Friday afternoon in May. Dark clouds were building off to the west as Buddy directed us through town and out toward the swamp on a narrow paved road that ran past several small farms strung out along the high ground. Beyond small pastures and planted fields, dark trees marked the edge of the swamp. The road was untraveled and straight, and I was going too fast. Ahead on the right I saw a herd of about twenty cows milling around in front of a house. The yard was shady, and the cows were looking for a cool spot. Almost at the moment I noticed them, they broke and began running toward the road. It took a second or two for me to see that the cattle were being driven out of the yard by three good-sized dogs of uncertain lineage. I was going too fast to stop and was too close to the cows anyway, so without touching the brakes, I pulled into the left lane. The confidence of the young is as frightening as it is misplaced. When they hit the blacktop, most of the cows avoided me by turning sharply to the right. I was set to pass them as I would have passed a slow-moving tractor. But one cow hadn't gotten the message. She was running as hard as she could, the dogs still following, and she never even tried to turn. My right headlight hit her just behind the left ear as she ran. The impact spun her around, and she bumped the side of the car and landed on the yellow line in the middle of the road.

I stopped, convinced that I was in serious trouble with the owner of the cow and with my parents, especially my mother. The cow was kicking and trying to get to her feet. By the time I got stopped and backed up near the cow, a man and a young girl were walking toward us from the house. I don't think either Buddy or Bill had said a word since the impact. Just before it, Bill, who was in the front seat, had stretched his arms against the dash and said calmly, "Oh, hell." I got out to face what I thought would be an indignant cattleman and said, "I'm sorry, sir. Is this your cow?" I pointed to the mortally injured animal in the road.

"No."

Before I could think to ask whose it was, an old Ford pickup painted with primer pulled off the road just behind my car.

"It's his'n," the first man said as I watched a man in overalls with tattoos on both arms and shoulders climb out of the truck. His hair was long and uncombed, and his boots were caked with mud. He put both hands in his back pockets and slowly circled the struggling animal. Then he looked straight at me.

"I'm sorry," I began again. "She ran out of that yard right in front of me. I couldn't stop. He says this is your cow." I lifted my chin toward the man standing with the young girl. The cow was bellowing and trying to stand.

"It ain't mine," the driver of the truck said and looked off into the trees.

I looked at Bill and Buddy hoping for some indication of what I should do next. No one seemed willing to claim ownership, and I was eager to go ahead and face trouble and get it over with. Bill was intently observing the cow's efforts to rise. Buddy grinned at me and said nothing.

"We need to find out who she belongs to," I said to the first man, whose tone and appearance were less intimidating to me.

He made no response, but walked to the pickup and lifted a sledgehammer out of the bed, stepped in front of the cow, and hit her hard between the eyes, swinging like a golfer. The hammer blow sounded solid, but I also heard something crack. The cow shuddered; all four legs went stiff for a moment, jerked, and then she sighed and everything relaxed. I noticed then that where my front fender had hit her behind her ear there was a hole in her skull the size of a baseball. The young girl knew what was happening as soon as the man reached for the mall. She started screaming at the top of her voice, "No, no!" And then, after the blow was struck, "Murderer! Murderer!" She ran into the road and grabbed the arm that held the hammer and shook it hard and continued to call the man a murderer. He ignored her as if she were not visible or audible and laid the sledge back in the truck. The truck driver bent over the cow and pulled a knife, and I watched in confusion as he slit the cow's throat and bright blood poured over the highway.

"What will happen to her?" I asked with the complete ignorance of a city boy. "Don't we need to find the owner?"

Both men were dragging the carcass onto the shoulder of the road, and the man who had bled the cow said with a slight grin that made me uneasy, "Highway Department will pick her up in a day or so. Don't you worry. You boys go on."

We went. I couldn't shake the feeling I had of leaving the scene of an accident. It was another four or five miles to the Gianellis' camp, and there I checked the damage to Mother's car. It was surprisingly slight. The right front headlight was broken. Plymouths had four headlights in the late fifties, and only one of the two on the right was broken. The headlight rim was a little deformed, but not much.

"That's easy to fix," Buddy said. "Your mother will never know it happened. We can get a headlight in the parts store in Picayune. We've got to go back for some groceries anyway. We can get there before they close if we go now." The way he said "your mother" made me angry because I felt childish.

The idea of not telling my parents about the cow had never occurred to me. It wasn't that I was too honest to consider it; but I had no notion of how to fix the headlight before I went home. Buddy seemed to know what he was talking about, and Bill was the sort who regularly took things apart and got them back together. Things were looking up.

We dumped our bags in the sleeping cabin and headed back to town. When we got to the place where I had hit the cow, we could see the big bloodstain on the road and the bloody swipe she left as she was dragged to the shoulder. But the cow was gone. It had been no more than an hour since we left. I was thinking that the Mississippi Highway Department must be a model of efficiency when Buddy started laughing.

"Those guys are over behind that barn right now cutting her up," he said. "I bet that one in the pickup owned that cow. Why else would he take care to bleed her? The other guy's probably his brother or something."

"But why wouldn't he claim it?" I asked. "I thought I was going to have to pay real money for that cow."

"Loose stock's illegal here," Buddy said. "It was his cow and his fault that you hit it. He was afraid you'd put the law on him. He'd have to pay you. So it looks like you were both scared." He laughed, and once more I felt stupid, embarrassed.

"Why didn't you say something and keep me from acting like an idiot?"

"You were doing fine," Buddy said. "Watching somebody squirm is always fun. You and that other fellow were putting on quite a show, each one trying to outsquirm the other: 'I'm so sorry.' 'No, it ain't my cow.'"

Bill and I had been friends for a long time, but I didn't know Buddy very well, and at that moment I didn't want to know him any better. I didn't like being observed with that kind of detachment. The idea of spending the weekend in the Honey Island Swamp with him had lost some appeal too, even if he did own a Single-Six.

We made it to the parts store just before it closed and bought a replacement headlight and went to the grocery store and bought baloney and peanut butter, milk and bread, and a couple of big bottles of orange juice and some eggs. Pearl River County was dry in 1958, but we had brought a couple of cases of beer from New Orleans. We went by the icehouse and bought two fifty-pound blocks. The camp had electricity, but Buddy's family still used an old wooden icebox lined with tin. A hundred pounds of ice wouldn't last that long in hot weather, but it was all the icebox held. We headed back to the swamp with enough daylight left to catch bait for the trotline.

Buddy's camp was about a mile off the main road. The fields on either side of a narrow lane were planted in tung trees, but the trees had been neglected, and weeds and blackberry thickets were reclaiming the fields.

"When he first bought this place, my old man used

to bust his ass picking up tung nuts and carrying them to Picayune," Buddy said. "If he made fifty bucks, he felt like a farmer. He talked all the time about being from a long line of farmers, but he built this place for a fishing camp. He wasn't any kind of farmer."

The road to the camp was little more than two tracks running between walls of briars, a jeep trail muddy and rutted.

"The bottom's pretty hard in all the mudholes," Buddy assured me. "Just don't slow down too much. Wouldn't do to get Mama's car stuck."

Tall grass between the tire tracks rasped the underside of the station wagon. At the end of the trail the road dipped sharply and broke out into a small clearing covered with oyster shells and gravel right on the edge of the swamp. Buddy's father had built two small board-and-batten cypress cabins up on pilings that would spare them from all but the worst floods. The pilings on the swamp side stood in the water. The cabins were little more than screened summer houses, but the corners were solid, and the sleeping cabin had wooden shutters that could be closed in cold weather. The other cabin was the kitchen equipped with the icebox and an old wood-burning stove. A porch off the kitchen had a long wooden table and an odd assortment of chairs and stools. Looking out into the swamp from the little cabins, I saw water, covered in places with a green carpet of duckweed, and tall cypress and tupelo trees draped in Spanish moss. Bass and bream were dimpling the surface of the water in all directions, and the late-afternoon chorus of frogs was getting loud. The sun was just going down, and already the edges of the swamp, sunk in shadow, were dark. Spending the night in a small boat in the swamp no longer struck me as glamorous adventure, and as I thought about the dead cow and the broken headlight and listened to the noises that came from every direction as the light waned, I wished I hadn't come along.

"Grab a pole and let's catch bait. After we catch enough for the lines, we can fry some for us." Buddy had already put the ice up and was ready to start fishing. "Don't throw any back," he added.

On the support beams under the sleeping cabin, there were five or six bamboo poles with hooks, split-shot sinkers, and corks. We used white bread for bait, rolling the dough into balls that fit onto the long-shanked number 10 hooks. In just a few minutes the three of us had caught ten or twelve small fish, not keepers if you intended to eat them, but a perfect size to bait the lines with. Buddy had also bought a big piece of liver at the store to use on the lines that we would run in the main part of the Pearl River. Liver was like candy to the catfish, he assured us.

Buddy's boat was a fourteen-foot V-hulled aluminum skiff from Sears, powered by a ten-horsepower blue Evinrude. His family kept the boat upside down and chained to a hackberry tree above high-water level. The motor was on a two-wheel dolly on the porch of the sleeping cabin. There were two gas cans that felt full. Buddy carried the motor without effort, and just before dark we got the boat into the water. After three or four pulls on the starter rope, the Evinrude coughed, puffed out a cloud of blue smoke, and caught. The camp was nearly a mile from the main channel of the Pearl, and almost at once the little cabins perched on the edge of the swamp disappeared as Buddy steered the boat through the flooded timber. I could discern no pattern to the route he followed and was alarmed to realize that I could not have found my way back to the camp if something happened to Buddy.

I wondered if Bill had any clearer notion of where we were. Sitting in the front of the boat, he seemed completely at ease. Buddy had the throttle nearly wide open, and we leaned hard right and left as he made sharp turns to avoid logs or stay in deep water, threading the way he knew through the trees. Now and then he miscalculated, and the boat ricocheted off a tree trunk or lifted high on one side to ride up over a cypress knee or stump just below the surface of the black water. I must have looked nervous, because when we'd hit a stump, Buddy would look at me and laugh. It wasn't the wild ride so much as the thought of shearing a pin that worried me, that and the fact that it was getting dark, and I had no idea where we were.

It was full dark when we ran out of the swamp into the river, and Bill and Buddy turned on their headlights, and the boat rocked gently as we idled along and our wake overtook us. I had brought a flashlight, but it seemed awkward and clumsy beside the bright and efficient headlights that left both hands free. I decided to leave my light in my tackle box. Off in the dark the waves we had caused slapped softly against the trees. There was no moon, and the lights from the headlamps kept our eyes from adjusting to the night. The world beyond the gunwales of the boat stayed pitch black. When lights hit the water, the river current was obvious and strong, and the water was mud-colored and opaque, unlike the clear black water back in the swamp. Above the sound of the engine I could hear tree frogs and locusts. Out in the river something heavy rolled and splashed near the surface.

"See any alligators?" I asked as calmly as I could.

"Not many out here in the main channel. Mostly they stay back off the river. Over your head, Bill," Buddy said as he nosed the boat toward the right bank.

Bill looked up and grabbed an overhanging branch that had a stout line tied to it. The line was weighted and hung taut in the current. Bill pulled in the line and handed the rusted treble hook to me in the middle of the boat.

"Bait her up," Buddy instructed as he tossed me the liver wrapped in butcher paper. The liver was whole, and I cut off about a one-inch cube and wedged it down onto two of the hooks.

"Stick another piece on that third hook."

I did. The liver was bloody and smelled strong. I leaned over to rinse my hands and thought about the long trip back to camp through the swamp.

As Bill dropped the baited hook back into the water, Buddy reversed the engine, backed away from the bank, and gunned us up river. We baited five or six more limb lines, all on the right bank, each one farther from that narrow gap in the trees where we'd come out into the river. I wondered if Buddy could find it again. It wasn't but about eight o'clock, but I was hungry and anxious to get back. It took some effort for me not to say so.

Heading back downstream, the light boat planed easily, and we were going fast. Buddy turned his headlight off, and Bill, sitting up front, left his on to light the way. After a few minutes Buddy turned hard left toward the bank, and before I could worry about crashing, we were cruising into the narrow cut that would take us back to the camp. I was relieved and impressed. Buddy knew the river. He seemed as confident and comfortable in the dark as people feel at noon in their own neighborhoods. We stopped on the way back and baited more lines with the small bream we had caught, hooking them on single hooks either through the eyes or just under the spine. The lines off the river were not heavily weighted, and the bait fish would be able to swim a little. There was no way for me to know whether we were getting closer to the cabins or not, but when we had set the last line, Buddy opened the throttle and we turned what seemed no more than one or two turns, and the boat slowed and scrunched to a stop on the oyster shells. Bill looked up, and in his headlight I saw the cabins.

We had not caught any bream of eating size, and so we each opened a beer and made baloney sandwiches with yellow mustard.

"I was pretty turned around out there," I confessed. "Running wide open through the trees must take a lot of practice," I added with admiration.

"Sh. . . ." Buddy tried to cuss, but with his mouth full of baloney and white bread what came out instead of a word were bits of food. He took a swallow of beer. "You ought to see the people who live out here fly through the swamp. There's this one old guy—my old man says his name's Bosarge or something—who stands up in the front of his jon boat with the outboard at the back wide open, and he steers through the trees by leaning hard left, hard right." Buddy stood up with his knees bent slightly and demonstrated leaning. "No hands. He's an old swamp rat. I guess he traps some, runs lines in the river. Got a beard and long stringy hair that blows out behind him. He looks like a wild man or somebody who's escaped."

"Have you seen him?" Bill asked.

"He passed me and my old man one night on our way to the river. We didn't hear him coming over the noise of our boat, and all of a sudden there he was. He almost ran over us. And he was running flat out in the dark, no headlight, nothing. He passed just off the edge of my light beam, but when I raised my head to follow him, my old man reached and knocked the light off my head. 'Don't shine that man. He don't like it.'"

"Why? I don't get it," I said.

"Old man said this guy was strange, half crazy. Lives way back off the river by himself and don't talk to anybody, don't like to be noticed. He's got no family, never goes to town. Tom Buck says he used to live around Santa Rosa, but even Buck don't know for sure. We're mostly here on weekends, but that time, for some reason, we were here during the week. That's probably the only reason we saw him. He didn't expect to see anybody on a Wednesday night, I guess. Old man said he might have killed a man once or maybe his wife. Hell, you could kill most of an army back in here, and they'd never find a trace. Parts of this swamp nobody's ever seen."

We ate a couple of more sandwiches and potato chips and drank a little more beer. I was thinking about sleep when Buddy said,

"Time to run 'em, boys."

We ran the swamp lines on our way to the river. It had been about two hours since we'd baited the last hook. The first two had not been touched and still had live bream on them. As we idled in to check the second line, Buddy shined his light up a narrow slough about twenty yards ahead.

"Benson, you were asking about alligators. Look over there."

In the beam of his light I saw nothing for a minute.

"Where?"

"Look right in front of that tall cypress knee there on the right," Bill said.

Two red points of light that looked to be three or four inches apart reflected on the surface of the water.

"Is that a gator?" I asked. The question sounded childish just when I wanted to sound casual and experienced.

"Yeah. A small one, maybe three to five feet," Buddy replied and grinned. "He won't hurt you."

"I'm not worried. Can you get any closer?"

"Not much, but let's see. I should have brought my pistol."

Buddy cut the engine and paddled quietly in the direction of the alligator. Bill and Buddy kept their headlights fixed on the glowing red eyes. When we were about ten feet away and could see the head clearly, the eyes sank beneath the surface without causing a ripple. They disappeared so quietly and so completely I almost doubted that I had seen them but for the open space the gator had left in the green mat of duckweed.

"There he goes," Buddy said, pointing just off the left side of the boat as if his finger were a gun barrel. "Bang," he said and moved his hand as if he had just fired a handgun. Under the water, but clearly visible in the bright beam, swam the small alligator, front and hind legs tucked neatly in, sweeping the water gracefully with its tail. It looked like it was smiling. I was not at all afraid and, for the first time, was glad I had come along. Nobody at school had seen an alligator outside of Audubon Park Zoo.

As we approached the next line, it was clear that something was hooked. The limb was pumping up and down, and the line was zigzagging back and forth. Bill hauled in the line hand over hand and pulled up a small long-nosed gar. The gar had swallowed the hook and was bleeding freely around its gills.

"Damn gar," Buddy said as he picked up the boat paddle.

"Hell, Buddy, just cut the line. Gars are tough. He'll survive and the hook will gradually dissolve." Bill was already looking through his tackle box for another hook and sinker.

"There's nothing wrong with my hook, except that

it's stuck in a damned gar," Buddy said, and taking the line in one hand he laid the gar's head over the gunwale and hit it repeatedly with the edge of the paddle. The blows reverberated against the aluminum hull, the sound carrying through the night air and silencing for a moment all frogs and locusts. Everything listened. Gars are ancient fish with scales on the dorsal side like armor. It takes a lot of pounding to kill even a small one, but Buddy was determined, even enthusiastic. As he hit the fish, the beam from his headlight jerked wildly across the darkness, and he paused briefly and took it off, looping the strap over the battery on his belt.

When the gar was mostly dead, Buddy cut out the hook and rebaited it without a word. He was perspiring heavily. The gar sank in the dark water, and as we started for the next line, I noticed that the water sloshing in the bottom of the boat was bloody. It was silly to be sentimental about a small gar, but Bill had probably been right, and something in Buddy's enthusiasm was unsettling. Conversation failed for a time, and we swung out into the river channel like three strangers on a bus.

Two of the lines in the river, the ones baited with liver, had good catfish on them. Each weighed three or four pounds. This was what we'd come for, and our mood brightened. Buddy unhooked and strung the first catfish as effortlessly as one would unhook a bass. He grabbed the slick fish so that the sharp dorsal and pectoral fins could not spine him and handed me the hook to rebait. I was nearest the line for the second fish and pulled him in and tried to hold him down with my foot because I was afraid of getting stuck. My tennis shoe would not hold the fish, and Buddy was impatient.

"Benson, pick the damned thing up and take the hook out. It's not dynamite—it's a fish."

I managed to get the hook out and lifted the fish by its lower jaw and handed it to Buddy, who grabbed the fish without looking and added it to the stringer. Again I'd been shown the clear line between being a novice and being the sort of tough guy I wanted to be and wondered if I'd ever be on the other side.

We ran the lines every few hours all night. Between runs we drank beer and skinned catfish. Around four in the morning Bill asked Buddy about his pistol.

"You got the Ruger with you?"

"Of course. It's in my duffle bag right now," he replied.

"I'll get it."

The Ruger single-six is a single-action .22-caliber revolver that looks like a cowboy pistol. I had read about them in hunting and gun magazines in the barbershop, but I'd never seen one. The screen door to the sleeping cabin slammed, and Buddy walked over to the table, drew the pistol from a brown leather holster, and laid it in front of us.

"It's not loaded," he said.

Bill had seen this pistol before and let me pick it up first. I opened the loading gate and tried to rotate the cylinder, but it would not move.

"Put it on half-cock," Buddy said.

I should have known. I drew the hammer back about halfway and felt it stop. The cylinder turned easily, and I noted that each of the six chambers was empty. It was a beautiful revolver, midnight blue steel and handsomely grained hardwood grips with a small Ruger medallion on each side. I felt its weight and raised my arm, settling the sights on a beer can about ten feet away. The trigger was smooth, and the hammer fell with a satisfying click.

"Nice," I said, trying not to show how envious I was, and handed the gun to Bill, who nonchalantly rolled the cylinder down his forearm like the movie cowboys did.

"Soon as it gets light," Buddy said, "we'll see what you can hit with it." He holstered the gun and laid it on the table with a box of .22 long rifles. "But right now we need to run those lines one more time. Grab a beer and let's go."

As we walked down to the boat, Bill raised his hand and pointed out into the dark.

"Listen."

We stood still side-by-side in the weak light from the bare light bulbs in the cabins, facing the immense dark of the Honey Island Swamp, black water at our feet and beyond the few trees close to the boat, darkness like a curtain drawn across the visible world. For a moment we heard nothing, and then I thought I heard an outboard motor, throttle wide open, way off, under the noise in our ears of mosquitoes and tree frogs. Bill heard it; Buddy said he didn't.

"You guys are just spooky," he said. "Let's go."

I still felt turned around every time we headed for the river. I could not have said with certainty that we ever followed the same route, but we did check the lines every time, and the individual lines and the limbs to which they were tied were starting to look familiar. I could imagine learning my way around. It would all make sense in daylight.

We were tired, and Buddy's reflexes were slowing down. A couple of times when he should have gone to the left of a big cypress tree, he went right, and in shallow water the motor labored at a high pitch, and clouds of mud bloomed off our stern. Once we ran solidly aground on a log, and all three of us climbed out of the boat into knee-deep water over soft mud. As we shoved the boat around the cypress knees and back to deeper water, one of my tennis shoes came off in the mud.

"Wait. I lost a shoe," I said as Buddy pulled the starter rope.

"Just take off the one you got left," he said. "We're not going back for one shoe. What size foot do you have?"

"Nine or nine-and-a-half."

"My old man's got some shoes back at the house that'll fit OK," Buddy said as he gunned the boat forward.

The night air was warm and heavy, and the water had felt warm too, but as we headed toward the river, I felt chilled in the wind we created. All I wanted to do was dry off and go to bed. Out in the river, it seemed a little less dark, and I was glad it was almost morning. We could go back and scramble some eggs and sleep all day if we wanted. That pleasant reverie distracted me completely when I was startled by Buddy's yelling. I turned and looked just as his foot slipped on the rear seat and he fell out of the boat into the strong current of the river. For the second or two he was under water, I saw his headlight blink and go out. He came up slapping water and cursing.

The motor was in neutral. Buddy had just pulled up to check one of the lines and had miscalculated our drift. As we floated away from the line, he had stood up on the seat and tried to reach the limb it was tied to. His foot had slipped as he leaned out.

"Dammit, Benson. Were you asleep or what?" Buddy said as he sputtered to the surface. "I told you to grab that line. Hand me the paddle."

Buddy and the boat were drifting more or less in the same direction, but his falling had shoved the boat away, and we had to maneuver a little to get close enough for him to reach the paddle. He used both arms to heave himself back into the boat as Bill and I leaned the other way. His legs kept kicking as if he were avoiding an invisible hand reaching for him from the river.

"Not very graceful," Bill joked.

"You looked like a big snapping turtle," I tried to join in.

"You bastards shut up," Buddy said as he put the boat in gear and headed downriver, tossing his head to get the wet hair out of his eyes. "I'll throw you both out and leave you. Don't think I wouldn't." He sounded like he meant it.

"Relax, Gianelli," Bill said. "It was funny. Nothing to get mad over."

"Just shut up then!" he yelled over the noise of the motor.

We went back through the swamp without speaking. Trees away from the boat were becoming visible, and I realized that Bill had turned off his headlight too. Everything looked different, the world no longer constricted to the beams of light we used to grope through the night. We put up a small group of wood ducks as we raced through the trees. I imagined they were making their eerie and beautiful alarm calls as they flew, but I could hear nothing but our noise. Where had the ducks been during the night, I wondered. Seeing was a great relief, but, though I was no longer afraid of the dark, the gray light impressed upon me again the trackless size of the swamp, and again I feared being lost. Water and trees stretched out of sight in all directions. Early morning light offered some comfort, but I remained uneasy.

Back at the cabins Buddy still seemed angry, and we unloaded the boat in silence. As we walked to the sleeping cabin, fatigue came over me like a weight. I didn't even follow Bill and Buddy up the steps to the porch, just sank down next to Mother's car. Buddy looked down at me from the top step and grinned.

"Your boy's about had all he can stand," he said to Bill and went inside laughing.

I was too tired to respond. Glancing at the broken headlight, I leaned back against a front tire and closed my eyes. I have no idea how long I slept, but I woke up with warm sun on one side of my face, the other side pressed into the gravel beside the car. I could feel the corrugated marks on my face. My right hand was asleep and useless; my neck was sore, and mosquitoes had bitten every bit of exposed skin, including eyelids, lips, and the soles of my feet. I stood up slowly, working my fingers to get some feeling back in my hand and pulled a tick off my neck. I could hear Bill snoring inside the cabin. I chipped some ice into a cup and walked down to the water. I saw in my reflection that the hair on one side of my head was matted and sticking almost straight up. I raked it down with my fingers. I heard Buddy holler something unintelligible in his sleep and heard the metal bunk squeak as he tossed. I wondered about the dreams of bullies.

Sitting on the edge of the swamp in the warm, still morning was pleasant. I watched sliders climbing onto stumps in the sunlight and saw a good-sized cottonmouth swim into the folded trunk of a cypress. Out in the swamp a pileated woodpecker clucked twice, then laughed loudly as he flew away, the wild sound diminishing to an echo. I remembered a boy in the scout troop I had joined when I was old enough telling me that you weren't lost if you didn't care where you were. With the cabins right behind me, I was comfortable, but I had to know where I was. Buddy's cabins were perched on the edge of big wilderness, and I had difficulty imagining the lives of people who lived in the swamp, people whose domestic arrangements included this wild and, to me, trackless world.

As I reached down to claw once again at the

itching bites on my feet, I saw that a small speckled king snake, alerted by my sudden movement, was making his way toward the water and had stopped a few feet away. At the same moment, I realized I had been hearing an outboard motor running wide open through the timber. I took my eyes off the snake and looked in the direction of the sound. It was getting closer, but I was having trouble coursing it. After a few minutes, I caught a glimpse of the silver line of a boat's wake catching the sunlight about seventy yards out. The trees were thick at that distance, and there were only a couple of breaks where I might actually be able to see, but I didn't really know where the breaks were and just tried to let my eyes get ahead of the wake and hoped. The boat would pass the cabins going away from the river. As my eyes raced right to try to catch the boat as it crossed a gap in the trees, I realized that I wanted desperately to see Bosarge. I had assumed it could only be Bosarge racing, no hands, with such confidence through the swamp. I never saw a person in the boat or even got a clear view of the boat itself. In less time than it took my mind to register what I saw, it was gone, the sound of his motor getting softer and fading altogether. Maybe he'd passed closer to the cabin than he'd meant to and turned sharply away when he caught himself, but the sound faded faster than it had come.

 I sat still looking toward the gaps in the trees until the spent wake of his boat lapped against the cabin's pilings, proof of the passage. At seventy yards without binoculars, it's hard to be precise about a figure that flashes and is gone, but my imagination had conjured him from the moment I heard the motor. In my mind I could see him standing alone in the front of his boat as Buddy had described him. I was aware of his wake chasing him. He almost passed completely in shadow, but then, a patch of sun, a white shirt and a shock of gray hair leaning hard left, and after, nothing but the soft swells of his wake. No one was ever less lost. I found a curious satisfaction in those images that were so vividly mine alone.

I had forgotten the king snake, but as I looked down, I saw that he had not moved. It was as if he'd been watching too. His head was up an inch or two, and his forked tongue was testing the air. His presence gave me confidence in what I'd imagined, as if the snake could corroborate my account. As I stood, the snake moved quickly away, but I reached down and scooped him up. Speckled king snakes are not aggressive. The ones I've caught have rarely tried to bite, and this small specimen was immediately docile and appeared content to be carried about. Bill and I enjoyed catching snakes, and I hollered as I went into the sleeping cabin.

"Bill, wake up. This little guy was just down by the boat," I said.

Bill was awake already, just lying in his bunk staring at the ceiling. He propped himself up on one elbow.

"Bring him over here."

"And that's not all," I said, intending to tell him I'd seen Bosarge.

I handed Bill the snake just as Buddy, disturbed by our voices, rolled over and opened his eyes. As soon as he saw the snake, his eyes widened, and he leaped from the bed.

"Is that a snake? Get, get that damned snake out of here. Are you crazy? That's a snake." His voice was quivering slightly and had gone up an octave.

"What's the matter, Buddy?" I said, taking the snake back from Bill. "It's just a king snake." I held the snake out in his direction so he could get a better look. I was enjoying his discomfort. Some swamper, I thought—he's afraid of a king snake.

"Don't come any closer." Buddy had actually backed up a step. "Get that damned thing out of the cabin. I hate snakes. I don't see how anybody could stand to touch one. Get it away."

"Hell, Gianelli, it's a king snake. Relax," Bill said.

"You guys are nuts. I kill every snake I see. Matter of fact, I'm going to kill that one." He pulled his eyes away from the snake and began yanking things out of his duffle bag. It suddenly dawned on me that he was looking for the pistol.

I moved toward the door, but Buddy heard me moving and thought I was chasing him with the snake. He bolted out of the door in front of me and bounded up the steps to the other cabin.

"I'll shoot the damned thing whether you're holding onto it or not."

Bill said calmly, "Get rid of it fast. Remember, he's got to load the pistol."

I ran down the steps and released the snake at the edge of the woods and watched as it quickly vanished under a bush.

The screen door slammed, and Buddy walked toward me with the Ruger in his right hand. It gave him confidence, and his gait had a little swagger. He was trying to smile.

"Where is it, snake-boy? Now you're not so interested in trying to scare me with that damned snake. What's the matter? Lost your nerve?" His voice was back to its normal pitch, but it was much too loud for conversation.

"It's gone," I said and walked past him to the sleeping cabin and found my clean clothes. "Let's head back this afternoon," I said to Bill. "I don't think I can stand another night with this guy. He's nuts."

"Buddy is OK. Apparently he's afraid of snakes."

"Apparently. Anyhow, I'm tired, and since I've got the wheels, I guess I have some influence here. How can you have a cabin in the middle of the swamp and fish all night and be afraid of a king snake?"

"I don't know," Bill replied. "I'm just glad the pistol wasn't in his bag and wasn't loaded."

We heard a shot, quickly followed by another, a pause, and then a third. Buddy was sitting down by the boat, elbows braced on knees, shooting turtles that were sunning themselves on logs and stumps out in the water. He fired six times and reloaded. He was a pretty good shot out to about forty yards, and we saw him hit four or five sliders. You could tell which ones he hit by the way they fell into the water. Farther than that he shot anyway. When he missed, we could hear the .22s skipping through the swamp like flat rocks. He was shooting toward the place where I had seen the boat pass. I wondered what Bosarge thought if he could hear the crack of the pistol.

"Come on," Bill said to me. "Let's load the car."

Bill and Buddy fixed Mother's broken headlight after we had loaded the car. In the daylight, it was almost impossible to see any damage, but for as long as she kept that car, the outside right headlight pointed an eccentric course, peering up to the right as if preparing for takeoff. Mother didn't drive much at night, and if she ever wondered about the odd beam, she kept it to herself. We had intended to stay through the weekend, but Buddy did not react one way or another to our decision to leave early. He acted as though nothing out of the ordinary had happened, and no one mentioned the snake. We tough guys, not quite defeated, went back to the city.

Three years later I was away at school when the government announced its seizure of approximately

140,000 acres in Hancock and Pearl River Counties in Mississippi to build the test facility for Saturn V rockets. Local inhabitants heard the news on a New Orleans radio station on All Saints' Day, 1961. Much of the land taken by the government was in the Honey Island Swamp, all wilderness in my mind. I was surprised to learn that whole towns where families had lived for generations were included in the displacement. NASA tore down homes, schools, stores, and churches in places called Logtown, Gainesville, Napoleon, and Santa Rosa. I read recently that Santa Rosa had been a hideout for pirates in the nineteenth century, and for the first time in more than forty years, I thought about Bosarge and remembered Buddy saying that he might have lived in Santa Rosa. I wondered if the swamp man I had so vividly imagined racing through the flooded timber alone and confident had listened to the radio when NASA announced its intentions. Thinking about the swamp I had seen as a boy, dark and mysterious, huge beyond my reckoning, its size alone intimidating even in memory, I guessed that Bosarge had taken no notice of the seizure. NASA said it needed all that land to protect local residents from the noise of testing the rockets. Their people put up some fencing and threatening official signs. But I also remembered Buddy saying, "Hell, you could kill most of an army back in here, and they'd never find a trace." Bosarge's claim to that swamp needed neither fence nor title. I bet the government men never caught a glimpse of him.

5. CHARACTERED BY MEMORY

> Thy gifts, thy tables, are within my brain
> Full character'd with lasting memory,
> Which shall above that idle rank remain
> Beyond all date, even to eternity.
>
> **(Shakespeare, Sonnet 122)**

In trying to understand my father, I have thought more and more about Powell, his older brother who died at my father's feet when they were both children. For most of my life I hardly thought of Powell. In his recent book on the sinking of the whale ship *Essex* in 1820 and the trials of the eight survivors, Nathaniel Philbrick writes that Owen Chase, the ship's first mate, "was plagued by what psychologists call a 'tormenting memory'—a common response to disasters. Forced to relive the trauma over and over again, the survivor finds larger, hidden forces operating through the incident." It's not enough, however, to say that my father lost his older brother when they were both children. My father saw his older brother decapitated in an abandoned gold mine in Colorado on a family vacation trip in 1914, his head caught between an iron railing and a rock outcropping as they rode an old platform elevator out of the mine. Nothing was ever the same. Even a phrase like *tormenting memory* seems a clinical and colorless description for the memories my father carried through the days of his life. The boy who would be my father learned early the transience of earthly happiness and stability, learned it intimately and irrevocably, and that knowledge affected everything from his reckless and self-destructive youth to his minute attention to the theory and practice of the law to his deep anxiety about being a father. That horrible moment and his painful encounter with a rattlesnake four years later made him the man I remember, a man reserved, stern, and solitary, a man who kept a tight rein on his feelings, but one capable of sudden anger. He never said so, but I am now convinced that he saw Powell's death as an avoidable accident, the result of horseplay and a moment's carelessness. He had seen it all, and the sense that things might have been otherwise haunted him. He owned a deep suspicion of spontaneity, stifled horseplay, and he conducted the business of daily living seriously, as if all our lives depended on his attention to detail.

 Many of the things I remember most fondly about my childhood are inseparable from recollections of my father's seriousness and caution, his formal manner and unbending will. I was fifteen or sixteen before I realized that other boys had learned and done similar things with their fathers in circumstances less burdened with care. When my brother and I were young boys, our father taught us to shoot a single-shot bolt-action .22 rifle that had been his father's. On occasional Sunday afternoons, we would take a sack of cans and drive out to the levee. Larry and I both liked to shoot glass bottles and burned-out light bulbs too. When you hit a glass target, the results are immediately gratifying if not spectacular, but you can only shoot glass once. Steel cans, on the other hand, can be shot again and again. It takes a lot of bottles to go through a box of .22 shorts. From time to time we were able to sneak a few bottles into the sack, but we always picked up our trash when we were finished, and Father did not like leaving the mess of broken glass.

No one in the late 1940s had thought of teaching firearm safety in a systematic way. Families did that sort of thing without encouragement from the state. Rifles, shotguns, and pistols were common tools in most houses, and fathers, uncles, and older brothers taught children responsible gun-handling along with all the other practical skills of ordinary living: how to drive a nail or patch a tire, sharpen a knife or the blades on a lawnmower reel, how to use an ax or bait a hook, and, if you got lucky, how to scale and gut a fish. You could get seriously hurt doing any of these things if you were clumsy or careless, but they were all things you needed to be able to do. Boys who admitted to ignorance or who demonstrated incompetence in any of these areas were regarded as odd, slow, and generally useless. My father taught us to shoot not because he expected riots or gang warfare or the end of the world, but because he had learned to shoot, and he understood the continuum of responsibility. He wanted to do the right thing, but it could not have been easy.

Single-shot rifles are good ones for small children. They are immediately safe upon firing, and our father held the box of bullets, giving each of us a single cartridge as we took turns loading and firing. Nothing had a warning label on it, but with our father around no labels were necessary. He had been sent to military school when very young, and his marksmanship was impressive. When Larry and I were finished shooting at cans at about twenty-five yards, Father would place a small matchbox or perhaps the empty box that had held the bullets on top of one of the cans and shoot it off. At school he had also learned the care and precision of military firing ranges, and his instruction concerning sight picture and squeezing rather than jerking the trigger was combined with safety lessons about opening the bolt to check the rifle to see whether or not it was loaded every time someone handed it to you, and about muzzle control, making certain that you did not allow the muzzle of the rifle, loaded or unloaded, to cross the body of another person or any object that was not a proper target downrange. I remember protesting once that because Larry had just fired and because it was a single-shot rifle, there was no reason to have to open the bolt until I was ready to load. Trying to argue my point, I turned toward my father, holding the empty but unchecked rifle about waist high. In an instant he took the rifle from me. I was not allowed to shoot again that day.

  We enjoyed these outings because we enjoyed his company as well as the shooting, but we knew that while what we were doing might be fun, it was not play. We were never tempted to think of a .22 rifle as a toy, and if our father ever sensed that we did not appreciate the seriousness of what we were doing, we picked up the cans, put the rifle in the trunk of the car, and went home at once, with no warning, no second chance. Some Sunday afternoons Father seemed relieved to have a reason to cut the session short, and I recall being puzzled and disappointed by those sudden stops. Lately I am surprised there weren't more of them.

  Some of my own boyhood experiences seemed to confirm the need for caution so deeply ingrained in my father's character. The family that lived across the street when I was a boy had two sons who were in college when my brother and I were around eight and five. Both young men were studying chemistry at Tulane, and they had set up in their garage a small but well-equipped lab. Larry and I had been over to see it a couple of times and had been excited by the exotic and efficient-looking beakers, the racks of test tubes. They had the first Bunsen burner I ever saw. Small children are all potential arsonists, and I was captivated by the burner. It was a fascinating place, and the young men who allowed us to visit seemed to us like adults, sensible, confident, careful. They let us look, but warned us, as adults would have warned, to be careful of this, not to touch that. They gave us a spectacular demonstration of the corrosive power of hydrochloric acid. They were a little strange, but we liked them.

One late July afternoon, my brother and I were playing in our back yard when we heard a great boom from across the street. We ran down the driveway to the front of the house and could hear screaming from the garage across the street. Mother came out onto the porch, and the three of us crossed the street and went around toward the lab. Several neighbors had arrived before us, and there was shouting that indicated both anger and fear mingled with constant screaming. I saw both young men led out of the garage and into the back door of their house. Both of their faces were bloody, as were their white shirts, and friends were holding bloody towels around the young men's hands. We learned later that they had been fooling around putting small amounts of sodium into water. One of them had lost two fingers, the other four, including one of his thumbs, and both had been cut by flying glass. One lost an eye. Larry and I lost interest in chemistry, and the neighbors had dismantled the lab before their sons recovered.

Around the Fourth of July a year or two later,

my family was spending a week on the Mississippi Gulf Coast. We were staying in the Edgewater Gulf Hotel. Fireworks were legal in Mississippi then, and my brother and I begged our parents to get some fireworks for the Fourth. The only incendiary devices we had ever been permitted were sparklers, and Larry and I thought ourselves too old for such childish diversion. We talked our parents into buying two packages of one-inch firecrackers, the ones that come tied together so that you can set off the whole string at one time. We went out to the seawall after supper on the Fourth just about dark. We lit a sparkler or two as a lead-in to the main event. There was no chance that we would be allowed to light an entire string of firecrackers, and my father was anxious that we learn how to light a firecracker without getting hurt, rifle-range care and precision once again.

I'm not entirely sure how it happened, but as we began our lesson in fireworks, I managed to light a firecracker and hold onto it until it went off in my hand. The best explanation I can give is that when my father talked, I listened. Paying close attention to his voice was something I had learned in my crib, and it wasn't until I was fifteen or so that it ever occurred to me not to. Somehow I lit a firecracker without anyone noticing just as my father began his instructions on how to light and when to throw. He began with, "Listen to me." I did. The instructions were, of course, mixed with cautionary matter, including a reference to the explosion that maimed our neighbors. I found the sound of my father's voice and the recollection of the explosion completely absorbing, and no sooner had the poor neighbors been mentioned than—BANG!—the one-incher blew, and I began to holler. Everyone jumped at the noise, and in the gathering dark I saw the color drain from my father's face. As he examined my hand, I felt his anger and his relief. I lost no fingers, and the burns were minor. We were forbidden all fireworks, including sparklers, forever.

On a few subjects, however, my father's sense of danger seemed off base even before I questioned it much. Having been bitten by a rattlesnake when he was twelve, my father hated and feared all snakes, and he tried for our own good to pass those sentiments on to Larry and me. Larry was indifferent to reptiles, but I developed a serious enthusiasm for herpetology. Father's fears appeared to be unfounded. I have captured poisonous snakes and have been fortunate enough to have done so without being bitten. I have received a number of nonvenomous bites through my own carelessness and the knowledge that such bites would be harmless. In high school, when I was trying to treat an ill-tempered Central American boa constrictor for canker mouth, I was very careful to avoid being bitten because the snake had large recurved teeth and badly infected gums. In summers at the Audubon Park Zoo, I had direct contact with a few very dangerous snakes without incident. But, while my experience with snakes seemed to discredit my father's sense of life's dark possibilities, at least one harmless snake put me in real danger. The snake was only a catalyst. The threat was LaBatt, a man who shared my father's loathing and who regarded violence against snakes and any who would defend them as reasonable. Killing the messenger was acceptable when the message was a snake. I never told my father this story.

In high school I had a summer job working for Louisiana Land and Exploration Company tailing chain on a surveying crew. One day at the company's dock in Houma, I caught a large black rat snake as he was going up the side of a live oak. Other members of the crew were amazed and incredulous, and I felt smug.

Once again my knowing a little bit about snakes and not fearing them had set me apart.

"Take dat snake and show it to LaBatt," C.J. said. "LaBatt love a snake, no kidding. He down to his barge over there. Take dat ting down there."

I was seventeen, and C.J. was one of the members of the crew I really liked and admired. He was the instrument man, young and handsome and deeply tanned from the life that kept him outside most of the year. It never occurred to me that I was being set up.

LaBatt operated a dragline barge for the company, and his barge was at the docks because the dragline needed repair. As I approached his barge and stepped onto it, I could see LaBatt's legs sticking out from under the dragline, could hear metal hitting metal, the sounds mixed with loud curses from LaBatt.

"Hey, LaBatt," I said in a lull in the noise. "Come see what I've got."

From under the dragline LaBatt recognized my voice and responded, "That you, Banson? What you got? I'm coming in a second."

I had known LaBatt for the past two summers. He was a friendly man full of stories, many of them about his son who had been a halfback at LSU. He also had stories of hunting and fishing in the marsh, and I had been a good listener. If asked I would have said that LaBatt was a friend, and nothing prepared me for what happened next.

He pushed himself out from under the huge crane that he maintained single-handedly. He was wearing khaki trousers and no shirt. His arms were heavy with muscle, his chest and belly broad and hairy. He was the color of leather. He was holding a large ball-peen hammer in his right hand.

"Les see what you got, Banson," he said as he wiped the sweat off his face with a red bandana, and he blinked rapidly as his eyes adjusted to the bright sunlight.

"She's a beauty, isn't she?" I said, holding up the snake.

LaBatt's expression went flat, and he raised the hammer in his right hand. "You get that sonofabitch off dis barge, now," he said and took a tentative step forward. He was obviously weighing in his mind whether he could get close enough to hit me without putting himself in jeopardy. His eyes darted from me to the snake. I was young and confident, and I had teased people who were afraid of snakes before, but there was something in LaBatt's bearing, something around his eyes that convinced me that if I stayed or tried to make a joke I would be badly hurt, perhaps—it flashed through my mind—even killed by that hammer. He surely was not afraid of me, and he had dealt with snakes all his life. In his eyes was no trace of what I would have called our friendship. I had betrayed that, and he looked at me as if he were seeing me for the first time. To my father, this would have been further evidence of the life-threatening situations snakes can create.

"I said *move*, boy. You and that damn snake get your ass away from me and off my barge," he said through clenched teeth and added an obscenity that to this day makes me wince about anybody who would touch a snake. His right hand was opening and closing on the shaft of the hammer, and sweat poured down his face. His eyes fixed on mine. I took a couple of steps backward, and when my feet felt the edge of the barge, I turned and leaped onto the dock and ran.

C.J. and Landry watched from a distance, and later they laughed at the fun they'd had. "Damn, man," C.J. said, "I don't know what's the matter wit LaBatt. He's always liked a snake, you know. You musta said somethin to scare him."

"You ran like a rabbit, Banson," Landry added. "You almos' found out what it's like getting hammered, huh. You did good to run like dat. LaBatt plenty pissed off you took dat snake on his barge." His laughter sounded like short little hisses through his front teeth.

Both men greatly enjoyed the joke at my expense and LaBatt's. C.J. admitted afterward that he knew what would happen.

"LaBatt hate a snake like no man I know," he said when he couldn't laugh anymore. "I don' know why, but he go kinda crazy wid a snake. I seen him swerve across traffic to hit a snake. You lucky he ain't had his gun." He paused and added: "But you sure ran off from there, didn't you?" He grinned broadly, as if he expected me to enjoy the joke too.

Several days later, at quitting time, I went back to LaBatt's barge and apologized for the snake. I told him that I had believed C.J. and that I was sorry. He had just finished restocking his refrigerator and was preparing to take the dragline into the marsh for ten days. He would be leaving before daylight in the morning. I stood on the dock to apologize, and LaBatt listened carefully although he would not look directly at me as I spoke. When I finished, he looked into my eyes for a moment, then let his eyes wander down the dock. He did not invite me onto the barge, and for a few minutes he said nothing. His voice was flat and without warmth or resentment when he said, "OK, Banson." That was it. He turned away and walked toward his sleeping quarters on the barge.

If you follow Bayou Lafourche down through Cut Off and Galliano and Golden Meadow, you come to the Gulf of Mexico, and Louisiana Highway 1 turns east across Caminada Pass to Grand Isle, where Barataria and Caminada Bays empty into open water. The island was then, much as it is today, a fishing village rather than a resort. Not many people from farther away than New Orleans go there. Late one summer my father planned a weekend fishing trip for the family. We were not going to charter a boat. My father planned for us to stand in the surf and fish for speckled trout. He had had good luck doing this at Grand Isle, and Larry and I imagined catching a whole stringer of silver trout, great fighters on light tackle and wonderful eating. Surf fishing combined two of my favorite activities: fishing and playing in the water. Mother was going to take her older sister, Charlotte, who was being crippled by multiple sclerosis. Nan Charlotte could still get around with either a cane or a walker in those days, but when she used the cane, which she preferred to do, somebody had to be there to steady her on the off side. She moved very slowly. Larry's and my boyish enthusiasms were tempered by having to support Charlotte, walk at her pace. She was a small woman, but her strength was failing her, and when she needed support, she was surprisingly heavy. She could not trust her legs, and within a year she would be in a wheelchair. The weather forecast was ordinary for south Louisiana in late summer: hot and humid with the likelihood of afternoon storms. In that line we got more than we bargained for.

  We were going to stay in two small cabins, each of which had a screened porch facing the Gulf. A boardwalk over marsh grass went to each one from a small parking area covered with oyster shells. In front the marsh grass thinned out onto a narrow beach directly on the water. We arrived too late to fish on Friday afternoon, but after we helped unload the car, Larry and I were permitted to play in the shallow surf. As we stood just where the surf was breaking and felt the sand being drawn seaward beneath our feet, Father told us yet again about the undertow and about how many careless and incompetent folk were drowned each year because they underestimated the power of the water. In the late afternoon that day, all of his caution seemed fully warranted. The surf was heavy and gray, and a strong southwest wind was blowing sand hard enough to sting our backs and legs. The horizon over the water was black with thunderclouds, and we could see lightning flashing in the center of the clouds. The wind was knocking the tops off of the whitecaps far out from the beach. We could smell the storm coming, mixing with the constant smell of marsh grass, saltwater, and an occasional whiff of dead fish. A big storm had formed quickly about two hundred miles to the southwest, but with no radio we had no idea of what was headed our way. Larry and I, exhilarated by the weather, ran up and down the beach, into the edge of the surf, laughing and kicking sand.

By suppertime the rain had started. It began the way thunderstorms frequently do. The wind picked up, and a few big drops of rain hit the screens and pocked the sand. Rain then came in windblown sheets, nearly horizontal, and it closed off our little cabins from the rest of the island, the rest of the world. At one point I looked out Larry's and my bedroom window and could not see the other cabin twenty yards away. It was, as far as we knew, just a big late-summer storm; but when Larry and I went to bed, our parents seemed distracted and uneasy. As I was falling to sleep, I heard my parents' voices as they were talking softly, but more quickly than usual, in another room. A few hours later, the bare overhead light came on, and my father was shaking me awake. It was dark, and the sound of the rain was covered by the wind howling around the cabins. One section of screen on the porch had blown loose and was drumming against the side of the cabin.

"Get your clothes on quickly, son," my father

said. "We've got to leave at once." I could not shake the sleep from my head, but I knew the voice well, and the tone carried a certainty that abrogated delay. Larry was already dressed. I was pulling on my pants when the lights flickered and went out. My father had not been to sleep. He was still in the clothes he had worn for the trip. We carried a few things to the car, but when he saw the water, Father said, "We'll come back for the rest of it. Go help Nan to the car. Go right now." Nan was always a good sport about her illness. Even years later in the nursing home when the disease had all but paralyzed her completely, she remained good-humored and cheerful. That night as the wind blew the rain straight across the boardwalk, Larry and I leaned into it as we helped Nan Charlotte from the cabin. We were all soaked to the skin, and Nan apologized for moving so slowly. We looked like drowned rats by the time we got to the car, and when we got her into the car, she looked at both of us and laughed.

The cabins were thirty or forty yards from the mark of high tide, but when we left, the water was under both cabins and ankle-deep around the car. There was water over the blacktop road down the center of the island, and through the water I remember seeing the yellow stripes that separated the two lanes. We saw one or two other cars. I do not know if we were among the last to leave or whether most people had decided that riding out the storm was safer than trying to flee. Though I had no sense of real danger at the time, we were lucky to be able to leave the island. My father seemed calm and moved us with deliberate speed and what I regarded as absolute confidence. Larry and I both sensed the seriousness of our situation and did as we were told without hesitation. Only when older and the father of two sons of my own did I understand the sheer strength of his will, a strength made more remarkable by his past. With other people depending upon him completely, two small children, his wife, and her crippled sister, his prayer must have been, "Please, not again."

One of the worst storms to hit the Louisiana coast was the Cheniere Caminada storm on the first day of October 1893. Newspaper reports say that on Cheniere Caminada Isle near Grand Isle, 780 people died. In 1893 they probably had no more warning than we had. Our storm in 1952 was only a minimal hurricane, but it had formed in less than twelve hours in the warm Gulf waters. In this day of constant coverage of tropical storms by an army of television meteorologists, it's salutary to remember that it has not always been so and that people in coastal villages have been surprised by violent storms from the beginning. Sunday after church, my father drove back to Grand Isle to retrieve the things we had left behind and to empty the icebox. Both cabins were still standing. The water had come to the top of the boardwalk, but had not gotten inside. Father told us that the cabin Larry and I had been in had been knocked off its block foundations on one side by an enormous driftwood log. The log was wedged beneath, and the cabin was listing seaward.

When Larry and I were around and needed looking after, my father never seemed to let his guard down, never appeared quite able to relax. He was watchful, always on duty. It was, therefore, both a surprise and a relief to find a letter that he had written to my mother, postmarked September 22, 1947. I came across it about four years ago as we were getting ready to move Mother for the last time. I think I know why she kept it all those years. He wrote to her after riding out the 1947 hurricane alone in our house in New Orleans. So much for me depends on my father's words, and some of those were tough and unbending. I have read this letter—the only one of his I have—many times, and I find in it a side of my father that I wish I'd known better as a child.

Off page one, along with a story from Buckingham Palace about Princess Elizabeth's plans for her wedding in November, on September 13, *The Times-Picayune* ran a story about a huge tropical hurricane with sustained winds of over 140 mph. The Associated Press reported that the storm, nameless as hurricanes were in those days, was centered about 170 miles north-northwest of St. Martin's or roughly 1250 miles east-southeast of Miami. The next day's report, still off the front page, put the storm approximately 800 miles from Miami. The weathermen were still predicting that the storm would turn to the north, but the weather bureau planned to issue "a preliminary hurricane alert" if that expected turn had not occurred "by noon tomorrow." The wire service reports all carried dates one day earlier than the date of the newspaper. The story I've just quoted from was in *The Times-Picayune* on Sunday, September 14; the AP report was from Miami on the 13th.

This was a big storm, and by Monday it was front-page news. The report, dated Sunday, placed the hurricane about 350 miles east of Nassau and declared that "one hurricane hunter airplane found conditions near the center 'too severe for the safe operation of aircraft.'" That same story noted that the storm had been discovered by a ship less than a week before, yet another reminder of the sort of information we depended on before satellites. On Tuesday the AP referred to it as "the great Atlantic hurricane," and the headline read "Lower Atlantic Coast Gets Hurricane Alert." The next day the storm had not made any appreciable turn to the north and was bearing down on Palm Beach and Miami. Conflicting reports now put the highest sustained winds at 100 mph and as high as 160 mph, the recorded wind speed at Abaco, an island in the Bahamas. Green Turtle Key was covered with storm waters two-feet deep. President Truman was aboard the *USS Missouri* on his way home from Brazil. Officers on the battleship were told that they might have to make a wide swing to the east to stay clear of the hurricane.

The Times-Picayune for Thursday the 18th reported that the storm had crossed Florida into the Gulf of Mexico. We did not see that paper because that morning my mother began driving Larry and me, her sister Charlotte and her two daughters to Washington, D.C., for my uncle's wedding. Driving from New Orleans to Washington in 1947 was a real adventure, hurricane or not. Mother did not want to drive through the mountains and chose a southern route through Mobile to Montgomery, across Georgia around Macon, and up the east side of the mountains. All the roads were then what today we would think of as country roads: narrow, two-lane strips through barely beaten back woods and swamps. All went directly through towns. Our top speed was around 50 mph. The trip would take about three days, but we were confident of finding clean motels at reasonable intervals. The car was, of course, not air-conditioned, and some motels were not, and the weather was hot, but I was glad to be going and hoped that we could stop one night in a motel with units shaped and painted to look like tepees.

The hurricane was southwest of Fort Myers, Florida, about 600 miles southeast of New Orleans. As we drove along the Mississippi Gulf Coast toward Mobile, the weather was sunny and humid. From Mobile to Montgomery on Highway 31, the traffic was heavier than any we'd encountered, and when we arrived late Thursday afternoon in the Alabama capital, there were no hotel rooms available anywhere. People from the coast had fled the storm and had occupied every available bed. Mother was weary from driving and put out by what she regarded as a plain act of cowardice on the part of the residents of lower Alabama. She thought it unseemly, I suspect, largely because she and her sister and four children had no place to sleep. I have no recollection of how arrangements were made, but we ended up spending the night in somebody's home in Montgomery. We might have lacked some conveniences in 1947, but that sort of consideration for strangers has gone the way of the dodo. We had no idea when we finally settled in and got to sleep where the hurricane would make landfall. Front-page headlines in *The Times-Picayune* for Friday, September 19, read, "City Expected to Feel Hurricane in Full Force By Mid-Morning," but we would not see a local paper for more than a week. For the rest of our trip to Washington we heard only sketchy stories, little better than rumor, but on Tuesday my father's letter arrived by special delivery. The first paragraph sounds breezy and casual, considering what he had just been through.

> *Adele, dearest,*
> *After waiting all day for your phone call that you all had arrived safely, it was sort of a disappointment to have to settle for a telegram. It came about twenty minutes ago. But, thanks to Providence, you made the trip safely and you and the children are all right. Your first telegram came after the storm Friday, about 4:30 pm—the first moment I stopped worrying about you all. I stopped worrying about our house and myself at about 10:30 am that day.*

The letter, which is fairly long, describes the approach of the storm and the preparations he made to ride it out. He recalled "gusts you could hear coming from a long way off" and big trees bending and "shedding foliage like confetti." "The winds," he wrote, "whined and howled all night, high up in the air," and in a sentence which I still puzzle over he described the gusts of wind getting "way up in the pictures for speed." The only pictures that come to mind are the ones which hung in our house, and the image of the wind in those pictures carries the sense of the storm being upon him directly and intimately, not just outside, but in the house with him.

Further on he describes a feature of this storm confirmed by the newspaper reports:

> *It looked very bad at about 10:20 am and I went into the bedroom and prayed—hard! And then a miracle seemed to happen. No sooner had I stopped praying than the whole storm stopped—literally dead still. The eye of the storm was passing over, but the wonder is that the dreaded "second half" never came! After an hour's lull, there were some fairly gusty winds for several hours, but not comparable with what had preceded the lull. Call it a coincidence, but it has all the earmarks of an answer to prayer.*

The city was spared the second half of the storm. The newspaper wrote of it as a storm without a tail. Once the eye of the hurricane passed over the city, the storm lost its punch, and the second half was much weaker.

The letter ends with a damage report and predictable cautions about checking on road and bridge conditions before driving home. My father closed with frank affection and concern for our safety on the drive back to New Orleans.

> *Baby, it surely is lonesome here without you and the boys, almost unbearably lonesome, but I thank God you left when you did, as I probably would have worried about you*

even more had you been here. Well, this letter is growing unusually long for an accustomed note-writer, so I'll close. Have fun at the wedding (which will occur before you get this). Keep yourself, Larry and Bob in good health and as soon as you can, after resting and visiting with Mama and Ruby, hurry home—carefully.

All my love,
Lawrence

The letter sounds in some ways just like my father. I can hear his voice in the damage report and the careful instruction about checking the highway conditions before deciding on which route to take home. "Baby, it surely is lonesome here without you and the boys, almost unbearably lonesome, but I thank God you left when you did, as I probably would have worried about you even more had you been here." Of course. When I read the letter the first time, those were the words that struck me with greatest force. The first use of the word *lonesome* sounds just like my father, plain but slightly guarded, but the repetition with the addition of *almost unbearably* marks true depth of feeling. The word *lonesome* has now lost some of its vigor—it has been trivialized by popular songs and general neglect. But it was a word I heard my father use more than once without a trace of irony or self-consciousness. The last half of the sentence is entirely honest and predictable in terms of his experience of family disasters. My father was always calm and decisive in bad situations, but he could not help expecting the worst, and even the careless and confident play of children reminded him of the contingency of all our lives. Living through the hurricane was easier for him alone. Combat veterans avoid situations that compel them to recall the horrors they witnessed. If they saw friends die, they may find friendship difficult among the living. Alone, my father did not have to worry about seeing another member of his family killed before his eyes. Lonesome he was.

The worst was never far from his mind, and all his life he worried more about us when we were there. He saw the tragic potential of every activity, and he did everything he could to protect my brother and me from the horror he had witnessed as a child. He even kept us from the rituals of mortality. Larry and I were never taken to funerals when we were growing up. Oddly, I don't think there were many deaths in the family. My father's father had stomach cancer in 1945, and spent most of his last days in our house. Our house was small, but Larry and I were rarely allowed to see him. We were told *No* when we asked. He's sleeping or he's not feeling well enough were the most frequent excuses offered. All we knew was that the house smelled strange. Three of my grandparents were dead by the time I was four, and neither Larry nor I went to any funerals. After that, no one close to us died for years. But I do remember that teachers or old people I knew from church—people I knew and liked—died, and when I asked about going to the funeral, my father simply said *No*. My great-uncle Andrew, who had been a missionary in China and whose rare visits I loved, died, and we were told *No* again. He who had been on hand for his older brother's death and burial did not want us to look at death so squarely. We could, in fact, scarcely say that we looked at it at all. My father had seen it all before he was nine years old, and he shouldered each new reminder of mortality without a whimper and did his best to keep the terrible secret from his family, to protect those he loved from all that he knew of loss.

Norman MacLean sought to console his grieving father for his younger son's violent death by assuring him that "you can love completely without complete understanding." His father, a Presbyterian minister, responded, "That I have known and preached." When I look at the photograph of my father at six or seven holding his older brother's hand, I remember that not only had his big brother died—my father saw him die and could do nothing to prevent or amend it. The bloody events of that day in 1914 were never far from his mind. That explains much of what he did for the rest of his seventy-five years and what he refused to do, all that he feared or suffered in silence, all that he would not allow or tolerate. Larry and I were occasionally frightened by our father and often perplexed as children, and even now some questions remain, but they are mostly trivial, matters of idle curiosity. Father carried his grief through all his years and ours. He bore it manfully, as one resigned to loss. I think sometimes he saw it as his calling, a mysterious vocation he could spare us only by absolute endurance. Perhaps it was, as such things may finally be, a gift. I wish I had understood. Our father has been dead now for twenty years, his old wound healed at last and his tears stopped forever.

A BEASTLY TEAR

From the start his sons called it hyena,
But when he coughed and winced once more in pain,
He sought precision then: "say hernia."
But they'd crack wise about the stirring beast,
Suggest a muzzle, visiting the vet.

Such manly teasing, though all good-natured,
Did nothing to relieve the straining bulge.
Some nights the daft brute refused to kennel,
Its wild ancestry granting no reprieve.

Afraid, hoping it might just wander off,
He waited four years to see the surgeon,
But it adopted him and hung around
As occasionally a beast will do

For bestial reasons no one can explain.
It stayed like some mad schoolmaster obsessed
To teach the way of sad flesh, brute cynic
Madly laughing in the gloom past firelight
Behind those crushing jaws.

6. CONTOURS OF HOME

Homesickness was a serious disorder for me, not just passing wistfulness. Lisa Knopp writes that "European medical men first diagnosed homesickness in the seventeenth century among Swiss peasants who had hired out as soldiers in foreign countries. For some of these mercenaries, homesickness was a fatal condition." There were times when I thought it might be fatal for me. As the word *nostalgia* suggests, it was regarded as an illness, but it is also part of the human condition, and some experience it beside their own hearth, surrounded by dear ones. It is homesickness that St. Augustine describes when he says, "My soul was created for Thee, O God, and it is restless til it find rest in Thee."

In some form or other, homesickness is rooted in our nature. Children experience it first when they go off to school or to summer camp. Older young men experience it as they go off to war or to train for war. Some boys appear to be immune to the malady, but many grown men sent off to military schools at thirteen or fourteen or even younger recall the loneliness and longing they could not hide though it shamed them. When he was nine, my father was sent to military school in part because he had survived the family vacation in Colorado and the accident that killed his older brother, Powell. His presence was too painful a reminder to my grandparents of their lost son, and for him homesickness mixed rejection and what must have seemed permanent loss. At Rugby Academy in New Orleans and later at Gulf Coast Military Academy he learned to smoke cigarettes and to fight his own battles. In those years he accepted an isolation from which he never fully emerged. More than once I remember hearing my father say that he would never send a child away to school. Without understanding the reasons for his conviction, I found comfort in those words.

Ordinary homesickness, longing for the familiar, the faces of loved ones, the assurances of place and routine, may indeed be a version of our deepest spiritual longings, but I have no clear understanding of my own inability to adjust nor why I so thoroughly distrusted change, feared absence. It may simply be that I was spoiled and had no real desire to grow up. I remember that I was often afraid as a child, but I have no words for what I feared. *Loss* sometimes seems precise. There was nothing remarkable about the daily routines of my childhood. My older brother, Larry, and I shared a bedroom. Mother put us to bed and sat beside each of us as we said our prayers. In the summertime she put rubbing alcohol on our legs and backs to cool us off so that we could get to sleep. From our bedroom we could see the lights in the living room where our parents talked and read after we had turned in. I recall being afraid of the dark, and many nights I kept my eyes open, fixed on the light from the other room until sleep took me. Our house was small, and if I woke in the night, in addition to small noises borne on the warm air,

I could hear lions roaring in Audubon Park, and nearer I could hear the regular breathing of every member of my family. Outside, amid the scurrying noises of insects and small nocturnal animals, the late choruses of tree frogs, were lions; inside, hearing my father and mother and brother sleeping peacefully, I felt safe.

During the day, I moved through a bright and stable world with nothing more threatening to fear than a playground bully, and yet I was afraid. I have started to think that I inherited fear from my father, though I never knew him to be afraid of anything or anyone, as surely as I inherited my mother's dark eyes. Somehow I seemed to have absorbed his abiding sense of the impermanence of all things dear. Perhaps such imprinting lacks reliable evidence, but his deep apprehension came to me in my crib. My father's childhood sorrow made him a solitary adult. Without being able to explain how, my response to what he had suffered was the opposite: I dreaded being alone. Through the distance of sixty years I am able to view my childish behavior with detachment. No doubt I was indulged, but when I try to imagine what was going through my mind the first time I tried to spend a night away from home, I am puzzled. I can only remember that my homesickness was urgent and painful and that I would have done anything to find relief. Homesickness was like gravity: it needed no explanation—it just was. Like gravity, it resisted me.

Andre Dubus once described himself as "a moving target for bullies." I knew what being such a target was like. Even leaving home for activities as ordinary as going to the movies with friends or choosing sides for a game of touch football occasionally filled me with an anxiety that was only relieved by returning. Young boys, susceptible to testosterone poisoning, but not yet fully symptomatic, are as xenophobic as savages and tend to regard even acquaintances as foes and rivals. Much of their warfare is symbolic, like the posturing of male elephant seals, depending on bearing and dress and size to intimidate. Within the circle of acquaintances, one always knew who was stronger, faster, and better coordinated, and the pecking order, once established, went unchallenged for years. Strangers from other schools or neighborhoods, knots of tough-looking kids with dark, slick hair and muscular arms, were a different matter. If you were not adept at reading body language or at sounding agreeable but not cowardly, you might be in for a real fight. Even real fights, in my experience, were pretty innocent by drive-by-shooting standards. The most dramatic results were usually no more serious than a bloody nose or a split lip. Rarely people lost teeth or suffered a broken nose. Switchblades and guns were still mostly movie props. Every boy I knew carried a pocketknife of some description, and many of the boys I grew up with had fired rifles and pistols, but that was hunting and recreation, and none of us would have considered going armed into the world. Even so, I tended to see all such potentially physical encounters as struggles of life and death from which I might never recover. I was not very good at posturing and must have had a look in my eyes that gave bullies confidence.

Because he was three years older, my brother Larry was not always around, but I had nothing to fear when he was. When we were children, boys his age had dubbed him Mother Benson, frequently shortened to Mother Ben, because of his solicitous care for me, the protection he offered against bullies, the assurances of home when we were away together. Dante writes that Virgil's saving him from a gang of demons was "like a mother, not like a companion," and so Larry seemed to me. Early I thought that home was wherever my brother was, and I have lately realized what an important part

Larry had in raising me. In his presence, wherever we were, I found domestic comfort and the reassurance essential to the idea of home. Larry had no intimidating swagger, but he was not afraid. Though he wore thick glasses (he was close to being legally blind without them) and had a bookish look, he was in every way tougher than I was. More than once in grammar school Larry defended me against the bullying of older boys. And more than once he fought for me and lost. He tried talking to boys who had shoved me around or punched my arm or teased me, but sweet reason has little currency in the schoolyard, and Larry did not think much about how a fight might turn out. Even as a boy his sense of the right and honorable action was strong, and his courage and determination won respect even in defeat. Boys who had bullied me and had beaten my brother did not want to have to fight him again.

Like all younger brothers, I wanted to do what Larry did. I wanted to be like him, but when I followed him to summer camp, my homesickness became his problem as well as mine. Before I was old enough to go, Larry went to Camp LeConte in the Smoky Mountains National Park near Elkmont, Tennessee, and he took to camping and hiking in those mountains as if they were activities he had been born for. The mountains of east Tennessee opened a new world to him, a world of great natural beauty that called him to adventure in the deep woods, a world that in some peculiar way felt like home. He loved it all: cool nights at midsummer, steep, wooded slopes and high ridges with standing timber older and bigger than any he'd seen, green shade cut by clear, cold streams that whispered their ancient secrets to him. He felt like some latter-day Bartram finding new wonders beyond each standing stone. He loved the camp itself with its rustic screened cabins and faintly military routine, the bugler blowing taps at lights out and reveille just after sunrise.

Counselors at Camp LeConte were a remarkable group, especially to young boys looking for heroes. Most were football players at universities in the southeast. Muscular and athletic, they seemed capable of superhuman feats of strength and agility. Many were famous in the evanescent fame of young sports heroes: all-conference linebackers, the S.E.C.'s leading rusher or leading tackler. All of them enjoyed their roles as counselors and as heroes. They were modest and good-natured, for the most part. Most were from small rural communities in the South, and, not much more than boys themselves, they showed great enthusiasm for hiking and canoeing, swimming and overnight camping, enthusiasm matched by self-assurance and skill. They were like much bigger and more widely experienced older brothers.

When his first summer at camp was over, Larry came home full of stories of things he had seen and done: a day hike to Laurel Falls, an overnight to Gregory's Bald or Mount LeConte, swimming and riding inner tubes in the cold racing waters of a pristine Little River. He said that when he first left for camp that his homesickness had been terrible. As he boarded the train in New Orleans that took him and several other boys and two counselors to Knoxville, he told our parents, "I feel as if I've been sentenced to Devil's Island." Years later I remember my mother and father talking about how bad Larry's declaration made them feel, how much they doubted themselves and what they were sending their son off to. But Larry's homesickness was temporary, and he quickly immersed himself in camp activities and forgot nostalgia. After taps in the evening, the bugler would go some distance from the cabins where the boys were falling asleep and play a few old melodies that sounded far away and drifted softly through the camp on the night air. The young bugler was perhaps a little lonely himself, thinking of the girl in Georgia he would not see for five more weeks. Larry said those faint serenades made him homesick for a while, but the wistfulness they stirred in him was also pleasurable.

Larry's report made everything about camp sound grand, and the next year, as he talked of going back again, I begged my parents to let me go too. I believe that I was ten that year, and I thought that I was as eager as Larry was, but the reality of camp life was not what I expected, and my homesickness, far from being a passing wistfulness, shadowed the whole summer and proved resistant to ordinary nostrums. I do not know what I expected. I may have thought that going to camp with Larry meant spending the summer with him, but we were assigned to cabins with boys of our own age, and there were days in which I never saw him. I felt betrayed by the ordinary arrangements of a boys' camp. I was certain I'd gotten the least appealing counselor in camp. He wasn't even a football player, and the boys in my cabin seemed an unattractive group of braggarts immune even to ordinary homesickness. On most days I saw Larry in the mess hall three times a day, but we could not sit together, and I wanted more of his time. I was unhappy, and Larry was my only substantial tie to the world I missed. Only in his presence could I be reassured, and so I made up reasons to seek him out during the day and tried to build my own counter-routine that would allow our paths to cross as frequently as I could manage it. It was a taxing and largely fruitless effort. Camp routine is deliberately structured to separate boys by age for various activities, and the people in charge at Camp LeConte did that efficiently. Years later I read a passage in *The Seven Storey Mountain* in which Merton describes his younger brother's sadness over such imposed separation: "The law written in his nature says that he must be with his elder brother, and do what he is doing: and he cannot understand why this law of love is being so wildly and unjustly violated in his case."

We were required to walk about 150 yards each night before lights out to go to the bathroom and brush our teeth. My walk from the junior cabins to the latrine took me by Larry's cabin, and every night I stopped on the steps of his cabin, toothbrush and paste in hand. Larry would stop what he was doing and go with me. Waiting on the steps, I could hear his friends saying, "Mother Ben, time to brush our teeth." "Oh, Mother Benson, Little Ben is waiting." I never gave a thought to how Larry must have felt about the attention I was insisting upon, but whatever he felt, he never failed to respond to my demand for attention. He never acted as if it were the burden, the obvious pain in the neck, it must have been. Night after night he shrugged off the teasing and walked with me to brush his teeth. I cherished those few minutes at day's end. Although I never said it, I rather liked thinking of Larry as Mother Ben.

Every week or two, all the campers gathered in a clearing across the river from the cabins for a bonfire. The evening was given over to storytelling, and the usual tellers were camp counselors or older campers. The stories were mostly ghost stories or gruesome local-color tales of axe murders and blood vengeance. The purpose was to terrify the younger boys, another peculiar rite of passage, a snipe hunt of sorts without all the running about. The older campers, veterans who had heard the stories before, made a great show of being frightened and of taking the stories seriously so that the younger boys would be properly impressed by the possibility of encountering homicidal maniacs escaped from the insane ward of the prison near Knoxville. These bloody-minded outlaws had murdered children in Gatlinburg and had eluded bloodhounds somewhere near Elkmont by wading the Little River, the very river whose rushing flow provided the background noise for the tale. I hated those gatherings because the stories really frightened me, and as I was about to forget the stories the counselors would plan another bonfire, and new grisly images would start me jumping at shadows once more. The only way for me to salvage such an evening was to sit with Larry. Discipline was lax on those evenings, and it was easy for me to edge around the circle of firelight until I found Larry. When I did, I felt that all would be well. "They're just stories," he would say. "Nothing to be frightened of. Just don't listen. Listen to the river, and think about something else." Sitting beside him, I could heed his advice. I could watch the storyteller as the firelight glowed upon his face and his huge shadow danced on the wall of dark trees at his back. In those circumstances I felt brave and grown-up, and for a while I took some pleasure in being off on an adventure away from home. Once I fell asleep reclining on his shoulder.

The remnants of old growth forest in the southern Appalachians, Christopher Camuto writes, are "the rarest kind of place in North America, a fragment of true forest." And of the trails leading into such places as remain, he writes:

> But the fragment of trail I'm on now jags through the woods as if it had a more intimate relationship with the terrain, unwinding footfall by footfall along a narrow bevel of least resistance

through the tangled vegetation and around sudden brows of rock without altering anything in its path. Unless you adjust your pace to match the jagged surface of real ground, this path will turn your ankle and run the toe of a boot into constant variation underfoot. A trace of ancient trial and error, a true trail makes choices that are sometimes hard to fathom, thoughtfully looping downslope to avoid a windthrow that disappeared a century ago but jamming you against the tree that fell last winter. It's the narrow, winding path of predator and prey, the way of hunters and warriors, lovers and medicine men. A rare thing now, a true trail, a trail that leads somewhere.

The Smokies, part of the ancient Unaka Mountain Range, continued to have a strong hold on Larry's imagination even after he stopped going to camp. He was haunted by a place and by his sense of a world coherent and undisturbed. He pored over topographical maps of the National Park and recalled the special beauty of places he had hiked to. His memories of Cove Mountain or Clingman's Dome or Thunderhead Mountain became still more precious to him in the flat, low land of our home. On rainy afternoons in New Orleans, Larry would spread his maps on the dining-room table. Though he tried to engage me in his imaginative amblings, I took no pleasure in such map work. I now know a little more about reading maps and have a deeper appreciation of them than I did, but visualizing the actual geography of a place by studying a flat map requires a trained imagination that I have never developed. The training, I think, begins by studying maps of places you have already visited or places that you know well for some other reason, but there is more to it than that. Such a talent requires a capacious memory for topological features and of mapping conventions so that you can transfer a sense of those places you know to places on the map you've never visited. The cartographer's craft is precise as such things go, but adventurous souls also find delight in the surprising imprecision and variation with which the natural world modifies the map. A few people seem to possess a visual imagination for topography. Gifted individuals look at a map and see the shape of the land, what the terrain would look like without trees, what sort of trees would dominate a ridge of a certain elevation at that latitude, what the vegetation would be like six hundred feet below such a ridge top. I think not all of this can be learned, but I do know that Larry was so gifted. He also had very good terrain maps to study. I was reminded recently (in an essay by Tom Kelly on turkey hunting) that the U. S. Geological Survey no longer publishes maps on a scale of an inch to the mile.

Larry had long wanted to hike the part of the Appalachian Trail that runs through the Great Smoky Mountains National Park, mostly following the Tennessee-North Carolina border, and one summer soon after we stopped going to camp, he convinced my parents to let three of us—Larry, a friend his age, and me—make this trek. Once the trip was agreed to, the maps came out and stayed out. Planning was as much a part of this adventure as the actual hike would be. As he studied the maps and noted the location of A-T shelters, he figured how many miles we ought to be able to cover in a day and talked about how rough a particular hike might prove based on the elevation changes indicated on the map. It delighted him to point out a waterfall that crosses the trail just here or the steep ascent to the Siler's Bald shelter right there—finger to map—a brief but steep ascent which required using your arms to pull up on saplings growing beside the trail. In his enthusiasm, which I did not share, his face colored with the warmth of both recollection and anticipation. He spoke rapidly and smiled between sentences as he looked from the map to me. He was trying to take me along. His return to the Smokies pleased him, and he wanted me to feel that excitement. It would be for him both adventure and homecoming. I was, in one sense, captured by his enthusiasm. I was dull and to me the map was a piece of paper traced border to border with incomprehensible lines. If there were essential information there, it was in a code that I could not read and had no interest in cracking. But I did most certainly want to be a member of this expedition and thought I was ready. The order and symmetry Larry found in his maps called him back to those deep woods and high mountain ridges, opening to his mind's eye all the details of that rugged country. It was as if he could see the trees and rocks themselves in the map spread before him. Going and planning were for him inseparable pleasures, and my lack of interest must have been disheartening.

Our parents were going to spend the time we were on the trail at the Wonderland Club Hotel, a rambling old frame structure just across the road from Camp LeConte. These were the only two independent commercial ventures inside the boundaries of the national park. Both the hotel and the camp had leases from the federal government because they were going concerns before the national park was established. Mother and Father would drop us off at the north end of the park near Davenport Gap and pick us up at Fontana Dam, down from Shuckstack Mountain at the southern end. The flu disrupted our plans. Two days before we were to set out, Larry got sick. He ran high fever and had upset stomach. His disappointment was obvious. Given the time constraints we were working under, doing the whole trail through the park became impossible. But in his desire to salvage something of the trip he had dreamed of, Larry proposed as he recovered his strength that we do the southern portion of the trail only, from Newfound Gap to Shuckstack, a three-day hike instead of seven. While still running fever, once again Larry began to pore over his maps. His eye was frequently drawn to the northern section, and he lamented the beautiful places we would not get to see. Looking carefully at the southern part, he was heartened by the glories we could anticipate. This hike through the park had become for him something of a quest, and though his original plan had been thwarted, the grail temporarily out of reach, he found pleasure and assurance in contemplating the hike we planned to make and in thinking of when he might have another opportunity to do the whole thing. I think I was secretly relieved. I was on no quest and had no intellectual or emotional stake in the enterprise. Three days of hiking suited me better than seven.

Larry recovered in a few days, and though he still felt washed out, we set off from Newfound Gap one cool June morning after saying goodbye to our parents and hearing yet again their concern for our welfare, our father's cautionary advice. Early morning mist gave to the forest we entered a ghostly quality that made me look over my shoulder to catch a last glimpse of our parents. The mist stayed with us most of the morning. The ancient forest was silent and seemed to take no notice of our passing. Once on the trail, Larry's strength returned quickly. Each of us was carrying external frame army-surplus packs loaded to about forty pounds. We taped strips of foam rubber to the shoulder straps to pad them. Freeze-dried food was not available, as far as we knew, and we had seen no way to avoid heavy items like canned peaches, Spam, and beef stew, all the comforts of home according to Larry, though we never ate such things at home. Boy Scout cooking kits and metal canteens also added weight. Giardia was not a threat we had heard of, and we counted on getting drinkable water on the trail. Larry had map and compass, knew how to use both, and we had nothing to fear.

Sickness had not finished with us yet, however, and not long after we had climbed Siler's Bald, I began to feel queasy. I convinced myself that I had caught what Larry had. Fifty-year-old memories are sometimes tricky, and I may have been sicker than I now recall, but at this distance I believe that I took full advantage of a slight indisposition. Shakespeare's Hotspur calls his father's cowardice before the Battle of Shrewsbury "an inward sickness" that "infects the lifeblood of our enterprise." My memory accuses me still. Larry's face knitted with concern for me, and he got out map and compass. We had done the twelve-mile hike to Siler's Bald faster than we imagined we would and planned to go on another ten or twelve miles to the shelter at Mount Thunderhead. It was early afternoon. Larry determined that we were just above the Little River watershed and that we could leave the trail, find one of the high feeder streams, and follow the water down to Elkmont where our parents could pick us up.

"Bob, look at this," he said pointing to the map. "We're right about here. If we drop off the trail back down here, we should run into the headwaters of Little River somewhere around here."

For him, looking at the map was like looking at a photograph: he could see our way down—rocks, trees, water, and finally trail. I knew nothing of watersheds, and the thin blue lines converging above Elkmont meant little, but Larry was confident that if we left the trail and struck off cross-country, found and followed one of the tiny streams that form Little River, we could reach a place in five or six miles where we could call our parents, assuming we could find a telephone. From the looks of the contour lines, some of the walking would be rougher than any we'd done, but the map also showed an old trail about halfway down that Larry guessed was the bed of a narrow-gauge railroad that loggers had used around 1900. If we found that, we were home free. Larry and I have recently talked about this adventure, and he believes that we came down at Buckeye Gap and found the Fish Camp Prong of Little River, but we did not know those names at the time. For us, in 1954, it was unknown territory.

To accommodate me, once again Larry put his quest on hold, and following his lead, we left the trail and started down. He never hesitated. Off the trail we hiked through beautiful wild country. Just below the escarpment, as we came around an enormous boulder, we surprised two sleek and quick black bears. These were impressive wild animals, unlike the beggars we'd seen on the roads in the park causing traffic jams. They ran from us with the grace and speed of startled deer. The way down was rougher than Larry had predicted. It took more than an hour of zigzagging downhill to find the first promising trickle of what would become a mountain river, and the old railroad bed was practically invisible. The forest had all but completely healed itself. Trail or no trail, we knew we had to stay with the water, but the banks of the stream were impenetrable with thickets of laurel and rhododendron, and the rivulet was not making enough noise to hear it twenty yards away. Chris Camuto has done a good bit of this sort of hiking, and writes eloquently both about what is required and what pleasure such walking affords:

Off-trail, I keep track of myself like a hunter, by staying aware of my relation to the stream and ridge that define the watershed I'm in. But in the field orienteering is an art, not a science. Not every creek you jump across shows as a blue line on the map, and some of the map's blue lines have run dry in the world. And in the southern Appalachians, laurel slicks or rhododendron-choked slopes tend to push you off your intended route in the way that a gusting crosswind affects a pilot. After two or three miles you may not be exactly where you think you are, which in good weather is one of the pleasures of walking cross-country.

More than once we walked in the stream itself over slick, moss-covered rock while ducking under interlaced branches of rhododendron. Our progress was very slow, and we were getting tired. We had good weather, but we were not taking any pleasure from our cross-country travel. When we stopped to rest, Larry checked his map and compass. He was responsible for getting us out, and he knew it. When he was satisfied that we were going roughly in the right direction, he would ask how I was feeling and urge us on.

Gradually the stream widened, and we found that we could stay close to it by listening to its rushing fall. It was a relief to stop fighting through heavy cover. The river noise provided comfort and reassurance, and shortly we came upon a well-used path that boosted our spirits and quickened our pace. It was after nine o'clock when we saw a light coming from the living room of a small house set in a little cove by itself, a steep, wooded ridge rising dark against the sky behind it. We had no idea whose house it was or what sort of reception late callers might receive, but we were tired, and the light shining in the dark wood seemed welcoming. Larry saw telephone lines going to the house. Yellow light shone across a wide porch that held two rocking chairs and several big ferns in pots. As we climbed the steps onto the porch, I let my pack slip from my shoulders even before Larry knocked on the door. I felt as if I had come to the house of an old friend. It felt like home. We had walked roughly twenty miles since daylight, and Larry had proven himself a reliable wilderness guide. He would have had reason to be proud at any age of bringing us out, but his accomplishment was all the more impressive for a boy of sixteen. My own part of our adventure was that of a self-indulgent thirteen-year-old still dependent on the competency and calm of Mother Ben.

When our mother died recently, she was the last member of the family living in New Orleans, and I was startled by the thought that in some sense I no longer had a hometown. She was ninety and living in the infirmary wing of a nursing home in New Orleans, a nursing home to which she had first come as a young girl with her father, who occasionally did evening devotions for the inmates. For several years Mother had suffered a variety of physical ills and an increasing dementia that some doctors insisted on calling Alzheimer's disease even though it was clear that she recognized members of her family even at the end. About six months before her death she had a stroke or some other medical event that took her power of speech. She continued to talk, but what came out was gibberish, a language without consistency of sound or syntax, without any point of correspondence to the English she had used elegantly for more than eighty years. She was the lone native speaker of her own unbreakable code, every sound a new coinage. She was like the last member of a tribe whose language would die with her. After a few weeks she regained some capacity to give one-word answers to direct questions, but she never had a real conversation again. She slept much of the time, as she suffered from congestive heart failure. When we visited, she would brighten and smile, then quickly doze off, wake periodically, struggle to say something, give up, and sleep again. In this way Mother followed my father without a word. Her death, I believe, was an escape back into language and old love.

In New Orleans people are buried above ground in tombs because the city is below sea level. Cemeteries there look like towns constituted of fancy dollhouses. The day of the funeral was hot and humid. The air was heavy and hard to breathe. The air-conditioning had kept the funeral home cold, and walking out into numbing heat and brilliant sunlight was disorienting. There was little shade in the cemetery around Mother's tomb, and the glare from white tombs in every direction made our eyes water. Mother was a small woman, and at her death she weighed less than one hundred pounds. Her pallbearers were her four grandsons, strong young men who lifted her coffin without effort to slide it into the space above Father. The head gravedigger was a heavyset black man in dark trousers and a starched white shirt. He had removed the marble plate from the front of the tomb before we arrived, and sweat poured from his face, darkening the collar of his white shirt. He had supervised a thousand entombments and was confident and quiet. His instructions to the pallbearers were delivered in low, even tones.

"Swing a little to your left, suh. Das right. Now lift the back end just a bit higher, so she come up level. Das good—now come on to me."

Everything in the undertaker's world is made to standard size, and there are not supposed to be critical variations. The top of Mother's coffin, however, was too tall for the space above my father. After two attempts which resulted in an audible bonk of wood against marble, the grave master signaled the pallbearers to lower the coffin, shook his head, and said with resignation, "Gentlemen, she ain't going to fit." It was an embarrassing mistake for the cemetery, and the abjectness of funeral directors caught in such a blunder is marvelous to witness. With much handwringing and repeated apologies, the young woman from the funeral home said that they would immediately move Mother's body into a coffin she was certain would fit. "Of course, there will be no additional charge," she assured us. Larry and I went back to the funeral home to watch what was done, and the rest of the family tried to find some shade while they waited in the heat. The transfer took about forty-five minutes, and the funeral went as planned from there. Mother, in an earlier day, would have enjoyed it all. She knew as well as anyone that all our earthly homes are temporary and inconvenient at best. "She ain't going to fit" can be said about any of them.

Over a lifetime the idea of home we had as children becomes the continuity of our memory, the tangible link to our past and to the living and the dead who are dear to us. Mother's death may have deprived me of my hometown, and the house Larry and I grew up in has long since passed into the hands of strangers. At this distance I confess to some embarrassment at the recollection of my childish nostalgia, but I know what it means to be attached to a place, and though the presumption of permanence is an illusion even for generations rooted to a spot, stable love is not.

At Mother's funeral the old patterns of our lives continued to play out: Larry was calm and reassuring, and I wept. Larry, retired from the practice of law, is now a Methodist preacher, and he preached at the funeral. As that familiar voice spoke the old formulas of consolation, I was reminded of all the times since our childhood that I have relied on his presence, taken comfort from his words. I saw the face I'd seen years ago poring over a map spread before him on our dining-room table. His voice was steady and his words warm, deliberate, and confident. The biblical text before him he found as revealing and reliable as a mile-to-the-inch topographical map, a compass whose magnetic needle pointed true north.

7. THE HEART'S SORROW

**Some branches sing when you put them in
the fire. Say I was one.**
     (Marc Hudson, "Wiglaf's Tale")

When Jim Kilgo died in December 2002, I had been afflicted for some weeks with a venous stasis ulcer on my left ankle, and I felt ancient. Jim and I are the same age—sixty-one—but I felt much older than that. I was old and bereft. Stasis ulcers are vivid reminders of earthly decay and the way of the flesh. This one had begun as a sharp and familiar pain on the inside of my left ankle. Two weeks before his brother Johnny called to tell Ruth and me that Jim was dead, the ulcer had broken the skin, revealing a dime-sized hole dark and deep into which my heart sank like a stone. Venous ulcers are not life-threatening, and my doctor assured me that they do not lead to amputations. Still, the pain they cause is sharp and severe most but not all of the time, and I felt wounded, like Philoctetes, with a mythic, unhealable hurt. In the company of healthy students and friends, I felt ashamed and unclean, though few knew the exact nature of my ailment. My wound and Jim's death made one aching sorrow.

John Glass drove me to Jim's funeral because I could not drive myself. I was gimping around with a cane at home and sitting down to teach, but driving to Athens was out of the question. I knew before I asked my doctor. John volunteered and I propped myself on the back seat of his Trooper and elevated my sore leg as best I could. On the way to Athens, John and I talked about Jim, about our own long friendship, about fishing, and about dying—its certainty, its proximity. The woolgathering of old men on their way to bury a friend.

A day or two later I recalled a dream that had recurred in the weeks following my cardiac bypass surgery several years ago. I was walking our yellow Lab on a familiar country road a mile or so from the house. It must have been summer, for I was in shirtsleeves, and the dog was panting heavily. A car pulled up beside me, and people whose faces I could not see shot me repeatedly. The shots that made no sound were fired from handguns in the front and back seats. Wounded, I lay bleeding in the ditch by the side of the road. The dog stayed with me and would not let the police or the EMTs near me until Ruth and our sons arrived. The dream had a peculiar cinematic quality to it, and it did not frighten or distress me much. A vascular surgeon, talking to my brother about bypass surgery, said, "Afterwards your body reacts as if you'd been in a knife fight and lost." That was only partially a joke and may have been one of the remote causes of my grisly dream. Another may have been the sudden intense pain that accompanies the dramatic removal of chest tubes following a bypass operation. That I remembered the dream after John and I had been to Jim's funeral surprised me a little. I felt as though I was losing another knife fight.

My lessons in mortality began early. In the summer of 1967, I was twenty-five, and Ruth and I had been married for three years. I was teaching English at Southeastern Louisiana College in Hammond, the town my father grew up in. John and Nancy Glass were in town for a visit, and I was teaching two classes in the summer school. One morning I went into the bathroom and pissed blood—not shockingly red blood, but dark enough, absent any discomfort, to be merely puzzling. I still had never thought that anything could be wrong with me, and so I said nothing and went off to teach. By midmorning I had a nagging pain in my back that was growing more severe, and by lunchtime I was in real pain. I could not get comfortable in any position, and the restless stirring about which pain encourages brought no relief. The pain caused by moving kidney stones has been frequently commented upon. It is severe enough to cause tough guys to fold up in the fetal position and weep. Dr. Richard Seltzer has elevated those who have had such pain to an elite among sufferers: "the fellowship of the stone."

Ruth called our doctor, and his nurse told her to bring me right over. I brought a urine sample, and when the doctor glanced at it, he gave me a shot of morphine immediately. I was, he said, having a kidney-stone attack, and he was going to send me to the hospital. It was my first kidney stone; it has not been the last. The morphine did not relieve the pain altogether, but for a time it no longer filled my consciousness. That afternoon I rode in an ambulance from Hammond to Ochsner Hospital in New Orleans. I cannot remember the ride at all. Ruth says that they drove very fast and used the siren occasionally. I'm sorry I missed it. When we arrived at the hospital, I had no idea that I would not set foot outside again for six weeks and that when I did I would walk out a changed man.

Those at the mercy of doctors soon learn bits of the language of disease. My stone was too large to pass on its own, and the doctors tried several times without success to reach around it with a cystoscope and pull it out with something they called a basket. Even drugged as I was through those days, it felt like they were using a bushel basket. Because the stone had caused some bleeding and because it blocked one ureter entirely, I developed an infection. Doctors prefer not to perform surgery in the presence of an active infection, but they believed they had no choice and cut the stone out. Medical progress, particularly the development of lithotripsy, has made the operation I had obsolete. One takes the science that's available and hopes for the best. I had no choice, and although I have lived with the consequences of that surgery for nearly thirty-five years, I have no complaints. The incision started in the middle of my abdomen two inches below my navel and went straight down approximately four inches. Following the operation, they did not completely close the incision, but left in a drain which would be removed later and which required frequent redressing.

The 1960s were certainly not the dark ages as far as the practice of medicine was concerned. I had a regular supply of morphine that the doctors denied me when it became apparent to everyone, myself included, that I was growing dependent upon it. After about five days I looked forward to the morphine shot more than I did to visitors. The doctors also knew that I needed to move around, get up and walk around the corridors, turn frequently in bed, and spend time sitting up. In other words, I needed to participate in my own recovery. But I was twenty-five, and my vanity had been more deeply wounded than my lower belly. I did not like the idea of walking the hospital halls pushing my IV tower and toting my catheter bag. Besides, I hurt, hurt in a way that shook my confidence in practically everything. I had played high-school football, chased girls, hunted and fished, and had roamed woods and city streets, as unaware of my health as a young animal, taking everything for granted. Having my tonsils removed when I was five and my appendix removed when I was sixteen were my only prior experiences with surgery, but they were nothing compared to this. This was real trouble, and I did not respond well. I sulked. I wanted morphine and wished to be left alone. Self-absorption is a powerful temptation for all who suffer. Pain demands attention, and painkilling drugs increase the desire for isolation. It takes all one's energy to outwit the pain or endure it, and the desire for ease is constant. Ruth and I had been regulars at church, but in my distress I deliberately avoided prayer and the consolations of faith. Prayer beyond the urgent petition that I get well at once was impossible, and even that simple petition became a challenge to the very idea of God. I did not walk as often or as far as the nurses wanted me to. I found lying more comfortable than sitting, and I felt terribly sorry for myself. In three or four days, I felt congested and began to cough up blood clots. Even as the blood clots showed up, one of my nurses accused me of malingering and told me in direct and unsentimental language to grow up. That woman has had a bad reputation in my family for years, but I have grown fond of her in retrospect. In some ways her diagnosis was on the mark. She knew unmanly behavior when she saw it.

For two or three days—I do not remember the time precisely—the doctors regarded the blood clots as symptoms of pneumonia, and I was given more antibiotics. The coughing and clot production continued, however, and a young urologist suggested finally that I have a lung scan. The scan involved an injection of some kind of dye followed by a long slow scan, some version, I guess, of a CAT scan. I was required to lie still, not moving a muscle, for over an hour. The scan revealed the blood clots to be pulmonary emboli, any one of which of sufficient size could have been fatal. This was a real emergency, and I was going to have another operation, immediately. I had been in the hospital nearly two weeks, and when they told me I was headed back to surgery, I cried. I was surrounded by people who loved me and who prayed for me daily, but I reacted to my condition as a child might. Having never been so seriously sick until now, I felt betrayed—the world had turned on me. Sooner or later it always does, of course. I had said as much to students, and I believed that it was true. I simply found the truth unacceptable. Some time after I got out of the hospital I was embarrassed more than contrite when I told a priest that I had not responded well to my suffering. After the second surgery I don't remember praying at all. His response was straightforward and double-edged. "You'll do better when it happens again." Not if: *when*.

Timing is important in medical history as in other things. I was to have the same operation, I was told, as Ben Hogan, the golfer, who produced pulmonary emboli following a bad automobile wreck. Saying that was meant to console me, but I was indifferent to the medical history of a stranger, even a famous one. The senior doctors all played down or failed to mention that they had never done this operation on a twenty-five-year-old, but a sincere young intern told me it was something he thought I should know. What no one could have told me was that in a few years, when President Nixon had the same problem, the procedure would be less dramatic, or that a few years after that clot-busting drugs like heparin would make this surgery obsolete. The daughter of close friends just had an embolus scare this year and had no surgery at all. She spent several days on heparin and several months on an oral blood thinner called Coumadin. Coumadin is warfarin, the anticoagulant in rat poison. Though heparin was discovered as an anticoagulant in 1916 and had been used as early as the 1930s by the pioneers in heart surgery, it was not presented to me as an option in 1967. Gordon Murray, a surgeon at the University of Toronto, made "pioneering contributions in the prophylactic use of heparin for the prevention of postoperative venous thrombosis," but I reckon heparin's use as a clot-dissolving drug was not fully understood, and for me prophylaxis was too late. Surgery was not presented as an option. It was a life-saving necessity.

Pulmonary emboli are blood clots that typically form in the lower extremities and travel through the veins back to the heart where, if they are small enough, they pass into the lungs and produce symptoms similar to those of pneumonia. Large enough, they can cause death by occluding one or more blood vessels in the heart and lungs. The inferior vena cava is the large vein that begins at the juncture of the iliac veins that return blood from the legs. Because pulmonary emboli present an immediate threat to the life of the patient, dramatic action is in order; and in 1967 that action was to ligate the inferior vena cava, thereby blocking for life the passage of deep-vein thromboses to the heart and lungs. Dr. John Blalock's reputation as a thoracic and vascular surgeon is still secure, and I remember him as a soft-spoken, kindly, and confident man who explained very quickly what he would do and what result he hoped for. The idea is simple. Ligate the inferior vena cava with a metal clip, and in time the body will adjust to that shock by using smaller veins to establish what is called collateral circulation. The blood would find new ways to get around the blockage and back to the heart and lungs. By the time Nixon needed similar surgery, doctors were inserting screens into the vena cava which would stop clots but would allow unclotted blood through. Screens are still used in special circumstances. Jim Kilgo got one put in a year before he died, but they were not available when I could have used one. Ligation stopped blood flow in the vena cava altogether and at once.

So much for simplicity. Dr. Blalock told me that following the surgery there would be some swelling in my legs, as my body responded to the shock and began to make adjustments. Nothing prepared me for what I saw when I regained full consciousness. My legs, tightly bound in Ace bandages to control swelling, were three or four times their normal size. The long, crescent-shaped incision on the right side of my abdomen, held together by heavy black stitching, bothered me not at all. My legs horrified me. They were huge, nearly without shape, and useless. I had to keep my feet above my heart for several days to prevent excessive edema. When I was encouraged to walk, I found my legs difficult to use properly, and even standing for a few minutes produced swelling that defied the compression of the elastic wraps. My legs were heavy and ill-suited to the rest of me.

My recollection of the summer of 1967 is spotty. Weeks in the hospital run together in a blur of bright lights burning through the night, days spent staring out at the summer's heat that rose in waves from the parking lot and nearby roofs. I remember legions of doctors, some pompous and aloof who had to be reminded where they were when they entered my room, and some full of generous sympathy and real warmth. Some were not much older than I was. Having been something of an amateur athlete, I went into the hospital with muscular arms and big, ropey veins that a child could have stuck a needle in. In six weeks various technicians and nurses with diverse competencies had drawn so much blood that my veins had collapsed and gone into hiding. I went in with ordinary legs marked with the scars of high-school football and a slightly more sinister-looking one, which I got when I failed to clear a three-strand barbed-wire fence, and after the ligation of my vena cava and several bouts of superficial phlebitis which damaged the one-way valves in my developing collateral circulation, I left with misshapen and strangely delicate appendages that made my clothes fit funny. Neither trousers nor shoes from my former life would do. About the time I left the hospital, dear Ruth, who had been at my side constantly, contracted spinal meningitis, probably in the hospital cafeteria, and nearly died herself. She was, in fact, in more real mortal danger than I was. She was pregnant and we lost the baby. We were kept apart for a hard two weeks. We were still twenty-five, but we both knew that time cannot accurately measure certain things and that we were no longer young. Contingency was real, and that summer changed us forever.

My mother and father were at the hospital almost as much as Ruth was. My brother and his wife were frequent visitors, and when Ruth got sick, her mother came down to New Orleans from Kentucky. During the six weeks in the hospital, I received two blood transfusions, and for several days after the second surgery my family believed I was dying. I ran a high fever that no one could explain, and though in some ways I seemed to be recovering from the operation, I was getting weaker and losing interest, inhabiting the strange and disconnected world which fevers create. One of my urologists asked my father to meet him at the hospital early one morning. My father told me years later that he went to that meeting expecting to hear the worst and that he and Ruth had prepared a list of questions for the doctor. The burden of the doctor's conversation was not as gloomy as expected, nor was it optimistic. My situation was quite serious, and they could not find any medical explanation for my failure to perk up. The last question on my family's list was, "What about that rash?" The immediate response was, "What rash?" The doctors came into my room and examined my forearms, my abdomen, and my back, instantly diagnosed a drug allergy and took me off of Keflex, an antibiotic which had been prescribed to prevent infection but which had caused the spiking fever and the rash. I began to improve quickly and left the hospital in a few days. That neither the doctors who looked at me daily nor the nurses who bathed me and rewrapped my legs had noted the rash is material for a cautionary tale that still gives me pause. Going to the hospital even for the simplest things is an adventure that can turn suddenly to misadventure.

I returned to my teaching duties that fall, moving awkwardly, like a new invalid. Except in my lower extremities, I had lost a lot of weight, and the collars of my dress shirts were two sizes too large. My proportions had changed, and though I was gradually getting used to seeing myself as I was, one of my colleagues burst into tears the first time she saw me. Other people's reactions to us are important whether we admit it or not. Gradually Dr. Blalock's assurances have become real. Collateral circulation develops more slowly than I imagined, but it does develop. Over the next year or so my body returned to a less outlandish form. Pants were still hard to buy, but that was in part owing to the bizarre fashions of the late 1960s. My figure was bulkier than anything the designers of clothing for anorexic hippies could accommodate. Khaki work pants were generally roomy and comfortable, so they became the staple item in my unfashionable wardrobe.

I was glad when I was allowed to move from wrapping my legs in Ace bandages to wearing knee-high anti-embolism stockings. Clothes fit better, and I felt slightly less conspicuous, less obviously Coke-bottle shaped. I was convinced that everyone could see the wraps right through my clothes. Gradually that summer receded; the stark edges of painful memory softened. For a time after leaving the hospital, I had a strong urge to go back and visit the doctors and nurses. I missed them as one misses loved ones and teachers upon whom one has been utterly dependent. I wanted to see them daily as I had for six weeks, to be reassured. It was a little silly, but I have also learned that impulse is common, and I have now felt that way more than once. In the spring of 1969 our son Robert was born, and we felt young again and well.

I cannot yet claim to have suffered greatly. The pageant of human misery on the evening news makes the sad ills of my flesh seem minor, and I know many brave souls who daily face graver challenges than I. Learning to be a father, going to graduate school, and teaching were all things I could do, have done with varying degrees of success. I was able to roughhouse with my sons (Andrew was born in Dallas in 1973), to play ball with them, not to be an invalid father. I did knock another kidney stone loose while bodysurfing on the Gulf Coast. The stones have caused periodic misery at unpredictable intervals, but I have been able to take my sons hunting and fishing. I still take long walks with Ruth and still make it to the woods to shoot at a duck or try to call up a wild turkey. Neither ducks nor turkeys have much to fear from me. Jack Shannon and I, friends for forty years, spend a lot of time planning hunting trips, some of which still materialize. Four years ago we both killed mature gobblers on the same day and have the pictures to prove it. Ten or twelve years after my operation, at Jim Kilgo's insistence, I was present for the draining of a farm pond in South Carolina and caught, with the help of one other man, a five-foot alligator. We slipped a noose over its head. The rest was close and muddy work, with much flailing about and falling down—in short, a lot of fun. I felt strong and capable, and I wanted to prove some things to myself. Alligator wrestling seemed a good way to do that. After a certain point I didn't think much about being infirm, and except for the swelling in my legs at the end of the day, I didn't need to.

When we moved to Sewanee in 1979, I joined the Sewanee Volunteer Fire Department and for several years was a reasonably reliable member of it. Because of its connection to the college, the department had two divisions, a student division and a community division. The student firemen were selected through a tough competitive process. They had their own chief, assistant chief, and chief engineer, and they were on duty through most of the academic year. SVFD is still the best fraternity on campus. On holidays and during the summers, the community was on duty. In those days it was easier to join the community division. Warm bodies were welcomed. Community and student firemen drilled together on Tuesday evenings. I took pride in doing all that the fire service required, all the things that younger and generally stronger men did. Answering the fire bell in the night is exciting, especially for one whose daily routine is academic, and fighting fire is strenuous and satisfying work.

Time began to catch up with me when I was in my early forties, however, and my legs began to repay years of inattention. I was no longer able to answer fire calls in the night without stopping to put on heavy support socks. I was later and later getting to the station. I was smoking in those days, mostly a pipe with occasional cigarettes and cigars, and I had several occurrences of superficial phlebitis in my legs, and because of impaired circulation in my legs, I suffered at least two stasis ulcers. Developing collateral circulation has turned into a lifelong process. I began taking Coumadin and wearing expensive custom-made compression stockings that fit like second skin, a nuisance to put on, but a salutary lesson in humility and a daily reminder of mortality. Exercise and compression are supposed to prevent stasis ulcers, but there are no guarantees, and at times I find it difficult not to dread the uncertain future. From time to time they recur.

One of the last calls I answered as a fireman was a rescue call. An undergraduate, one of my former students, had fallen off a cliff and broken his back. The call came in about midnight, and I ended up being taken to the hospital along with the injured young man. The rescue was strenuous, and when we had gotten him back to the top, I was breathless and my heart was racing and out of rhythm. I had a cardiac arrhythmia called atrial fibrillation, an electrical problem. While it is not directly life-threatening, patients with atrial fibrillation are seven times more likely than normal folk to suffer strokes. It is customary to prescribe Coumadin to lessen the likelihood of a stroke, and I was fortunate to have been taking that blood thinner already. Some people with atrial fib are unaware of it; others can feel the irregularity and occasionally experience some discomfort from it. I was aware of mine much of the time, and I now and then felt hollow chested, breathless, and weak. Dr. Joseph Fredi, my cardiologist, who did not seem overly concerned by the symptoms I vaguely described, suggested in the fall of 1998 that I have a cardiac stress test on a treadmill. Doctors must have a set of canned responses that they save for schoolteachers. In his essay on having cardiac bypass surgery, Joseph Epstein writes that the doctor monitoring his stress test said at the end, "I'm sorry, but you failed the test." That's eerily close to what I was told. Holding one end the EKG strip in his left hand, the doctor said, "If I had to grade this paper, I'd give it an F."

When his cardiologist decided that my father should have an angiogram, his heart was already too weak. The doctor halted the procedure almost as soon as it started. Scheduling an angiogram, however, did not strike me as a drastic matter. I was convinced that there was nothing seriously wrong, but Jack and Jan Shannon drove up from Birmingham to Nashville, and I began to wonder if I were missing something. Dr. Fredi did the angiogram, and when he came to see me in the recovery room, he had a pleasant-looking young man in tow. Dr. Fredi introduced the young doctor by saying, "Dr. Benson, this is Dr. Shuman. He's going to do your surgery. What I saw were three blocked arteries, and you need to have a triple bypass."

I reacted slowly to that news. I remember being struck particularly by how young Dr. Shuman looked. I wanted to say something smart-alecky about children practicing medicine, but I lost the thread of my thought. When I got my wits back, I said, "Well, can we do it next summer?" It was the end of October, and the semester was just a little more than half over.

Both doctors smiled indulgently, and Dr. Fredi told me that he did not want to wait. I proposed the long Christmas holiday, and he shook his head. "Dr. Shuman can do your surgery in the morning. It's important to go ahead."

It was my turn to object. "That's simply not possible," I heard myself say. "I need to inform the dean. I need to get somebody to cover my classes. I can't just not show up tomorrow." It all sounded reasonable to me.

"What do you teach?" Dr. Shuman asked.

"Chaucer."

Both doctors smiled. "It's harder to find someone to teach Chaucer than it is to find a surgeon to do a bypass," Dr. Shuman said to Dr. Fredi. I had a week. But in fact Chaucer alone had not bought me that week. Because I take Coumadin, I needed to get that blood thinner out of my system before surgery. I have a protein-S deficiency, however, and tend to form blood clots more readily than most, and as I stopped taking Coumadin and made arrangements for my classes, I was taught to give myself injections of Lovenox, an anticoagulant that stays in the body for only about eight hours. For the week before surgery I stuck my abdomen with a short needle morning and evening. I asked Dr. Fredi if the surgery were an event for which we ought to call the children home. "Oh, yes," he replied without hesitation.

The evening before surgery I made my confession and received the Sacrament, and Ruth and Robert and Andrew and I went out to dinner. Robert had come from culinary school in Oregon and Andrew, newly married, from Georgia. It was good to have the boys around, and we had a pleasant evening, avoiding conversation about my health and what lay ahead. They were all solicitous, and it is unnerving to recall the appeal sickness can have for the self-centered. I frankly enjoyed being the center of attention, and I had little thought for the surgery. I claim no sanctity, and I do not think of myself as a person of great courage, but I was not anxious about the next morning. I had done all that a Christian ought to do when facing heart surgery, and my dear family, being themselves, were giving me their courage. Back at the hospital, we all watched a video on bypass surgery and joked about the quality of educational film.

St. Thomas Hospital is generous with families, and the next morning, as I was being prepared, Ruth and Robert and Andrew were present. While I was being scrubbed and shaved and having blood drawn and IVs inserted, those loved faces were hovering near the bed, holding my hands and making small but precious talk. Ruth named friends who had gathered in the waiting room to keep her company and others who were waiting by telephones to offer their love. As I waited to be wheeled into surgery, I had a clear sense of being surrounded by a cloud of witnesses, a cloud that I imagined included the living and the dead. Their names are an essential catalogue in my recollections though I never saw them assembled in one place.

When I went home, my brother, Larry, came and stayed a week, and we all enjoyed a week of Robert's cooking. Immediately following bypass surgery, the liver produces no cholesterol, and for a while heart patients can eat anything. The catch is that I didn't have much of an appetite, but I tried to eat as much as I could of the good things I knew that I was soon to be forbidden. This was not the first time I had been surrounded by such a cloud of witnesses, but, unlike my response to my earlier encounter with serious illness, this time I felt no resentment, no temptation to withdraw. I was full of hope and gratitude. My father had thought that his health and Mother's were nobody else's damned business. He seemed determined to suffer alone. Healing or not he knew was God's business, but he moved forward by the sheer force of will into whatever lay ahead.

Of the surgery itself, of course, I have no recollection. I have read Dr. Shuman's description of my operation, but the precise and bloodless language of that report seems distant and impersonal. He could have been describing anyone's surgery.

> A right internal jugular Swan-Ganz catheter and left radial arterial line were placed. After the induction of general anesthesia, the patient was prepped and draped in the usual sterile fashion. Standard median sternotomy incision was made with the incision extended down through the subcutaneous tissue. The sternum was opened with the use of the sternal saw.

The report never uses the graphic slang that describes this as *cracking a chest*. A few sentences later: "Antegrade cardioplegia was infused in the aortic root with rapid myocardial cooling and cardiac arrest." I read without emotion that my heart stopped. What does strike me is the spare eloquence used to describe this violent and mortal matter. It's all in a day's work for a man with the nerves of a Navy pilot—no syllable of hesitation, no hint of self-doubt. "The sternum was reapproximated with stainless steel wires." The word *reapproximated* is used precisely, but it contains a trace of the artistic dimension of the surgeon's skill.

What I do remember was largely uneventful. When I woke up in the cardiac intensive-care unit, I was connected to various monitors and had tubes stuck in nearly every conceivable place: a urinary catheter, I.V.s in both arms, a central or arterial line, and, as I had been warned, an intratracheal tube that made it impossible to speak. I did not panic as some patients do when they become aware of the tube in their throats, but it is uncomfortable and somewhat alarming. I understood at least the impulse to remove it myself. My first recollections upon waking were of being hovered over by a solicitous and confident young woman and the faces of Ruth, Robert, and Andrew. I was greatly relieved by the removal of the intratracheal tube, but my voice was weak. Andrew said that I sounded like Marlon Brando in *Godfather*. The nurse brought Ruth and the boys back to my bedside, saying, "You guys come over here and visit." I have never cared for the modern and almost universal use of the term *guys* applied to both sexes, and my first words after surgery were a correction: "She's not a guy." The nurse shrugged it off with a laugh, and Robert said, "I see they didn't remove your curmudgeon gland."

On two occasions after surgery my blood pressure dropped low enough to alarm the doctors. Low blood pressure does not hurt, however, and I felt too weak to be much concerned by my condition. There was some uncertainty about the causes of my blood pressure drop, but at least one of the possibilities was internal bleeding, and I remember Dr. Fredi saying that if they tried something—I've forgotten what exactly—to raise my blood pressure that did not work, I would have to go back to surgery. Remembering the summer of 1967 in New Orleans, I thought, *Here we go again*, but even the thought of having my chest opened twice in as many days did not affect me much. Whatever they tried worked, and I was spared a second surgery. I was also spared the painful cutting of one's leg to harvest the vessels that are generally used to bypass the blockages. Because of my vena cava ligation, the veins in my legs were not useful, and Dr. Shuman harvested both of my mammary arteries from my chest wall. No additional incision was necessary, but because the arteries have to be teased out of the muscles of the chest, there is some additional lingering discomfort in the chest wall, but it is minor compared the violence of having one's chest cracked.

No one tells you about chest tubes. Following bypass surgery, there are tubes, in my case three of them, left in the chest and attached to a pump which draws off fluids that are a natural result of cardiac surgery. The doctors watch the tubes with serious interest. Too much blood from the chest tubes indicates a problem. I've forgotten how long my chest tubes were in—three or four days perhaps—but the worst pain I experienced during the entire hospital stay was when Dr. Shuman took all three chest tubes in his right hand and with the same movement a magician uses to remove a rabbit from his hat, but without saying *Presto!*, jerked the tubes out. It happened very quickly and hurt like hell. I felt the tubes move deep in my chest and realized what sensible people have perhaps always known: that there are pain sensors inside. I had an inkling then of what a knife or bullet wound might feel like.

Atrial fibrillation is not corrected by a bypass, and about a year after that surgery, somewhat anticlimactically, Dr. Shuman installed a pacemaker in my chest. Without it, my heart rate occasionally and suddenly dropped to around thirty beats per minute. Passing out was a real possibility.

All of my memories of disease and trauma are crowded with images of family and friends. From 1967 I remember the faces of my mother and father living through what they believed might be their younger son's last days. My father, no stranger to grief, was trying to attend to details and stay calm, but he was also pulling away, withdrawing as his dark history compelled him, moving him from us even as he drove Mother and Ruth back and forth to the hospital. In 1998 I remember Jack and Jan coming to Nashville, first for the angiogram and then coming back a week later for the main event. And Robert and Andrew dropped everything and came when we called. I still feel the warmth of their strong fingers holding mine. And always there was Ruth, whose constancy and strength in trial—for better or for worse—I have depended upon. Those dear faces and others crowd out the pain which I cannot now remember. My father's childhood sorrow isolated him. My trials have had the opposite effect. They have taught me the obvious lessons of transience and mortality, but they have also revealed the power of love, the durable bonds of domestic affection, the generosity of friendship, and all I know of *caritas*.

My father has been dead for more than twenty years, and at sixty-four I still find myself wondering how he might have reacted to certain events. In writing this account of my medical adventures, he has most insistently occupied my thoughts. Because he hated and feared all snakes, poisonous or not, seeing snakes always brings to mind my father and the burden he carried. Yesterday morning at first light I took the dog outside, and we encountered a large black rat snake on the deck. Samson has had no experience with snakes, and I let him approach this nonvenomous one just to see what he would do. The snake, surprised by the dog, did exactly what I thought it would: it threw the front third of its length into a defensive striking coil, its tail soundlessly twitching. Samson was unsure of his role in this drama and simply presented his nose to be bitten. The snake hesitated a moment, and I called Samson to me, disappointed by his lack of caution. Had the snake been poisonous, Samson might have been in real trouble. Our old yellow Lab, Jessie, seemed to have been born with the wit to give snakes a wide berth. She had, in fact, a distinctive bark which she used only for snakes. The year before she died, Jessie found a copperhead on the driveway and alerted us to its presence with an insistent high-pitched bark. Samson has no such native wit. With the dog gone, the snake gradually relaxed and moved deliberately back under the deck. It was for me a pleasant way to begin the morning. There have been more snakes around this summer than usual, or at least we've seen more. There was a young milk snake dead on the road in front of our house the other day. Folks down the street with small children have killed two copperheads recently, and a week or so ago our neighbors, a retired couple, called the police to dispatch a 51-inch female timber rattler that was sunning on their driveway. The officer who killed the snake planned to eat it.

Back in the house, I thought how different my reaction to our morning encounter was from what my father's would have been. The presence of snakes, even poisonous ones, helps bring the world to life for me. Just knowing they're around brings clarity and consolation to a life mostly separated from wild nature, a stay against confusion. Because he had been bitten by a rattlesnake when he was twelve, seeing a snake on his deck first thing in the morning would have ruined my father's day and several of the mornings that followed. Despite our differences on this subject, my own experience, with important exceptions, still takes its shape from his. Things make sense or fail to make sense in terms he first laid out. The grim events of his childhood—his snakebite and his brother's accidental death—marked his character, but they also affected the kind of husband and father I became, though it has taken me more than thirty years to see it.

The dark moments of my father's boyhood are precise and datable, and, of course, he never forgot. Philoctetes inherited the great bow of Heracles, but on his way to Troy he was bitten by a poisonous snake. The snakebite became a "suppurating and malodorous" wound that would not heal, and his companions abandoned him on Lemnos. Odysseus explains, "All the camp was haunted by him." Fundamental for Edmund Wilson in this story is "the conception of superior strength as inseparable from disability." Near the end of the *Philoctetes* Sophocles has Heracles address these words to his snakebit protagonist:

> Let me reveal to you my own story first,
> let me show the tasks and sufferings that were mine,
> and, at the last, the winning of deathless merit.
> All this you can see in me now.
> All this must be your suffering too,
> the winning of a life to an end in glory,
> out of this suffering.

My father's story does, of course, come first, but finally it merges with my own. He could not have foreseen the ways in which his sorrow and pain gradually shadowed others' years. I had no reason like my father's to be quick-tempered and stern with my sons. I did simply what I thought fathers did. My severity lacked the iron conviction of his, however, and much of what I did seems merely quixotic to me now and was doubtless confusing to the boys. When they were young, I knew something of contingency, and I was an apprehensive parent. I was afraid for my children before either of them gave me reason to fear. But neither my father's sorrow nor its dark train has the final word. Both of us were wounded, by heartbreaking accident or by illness, but in reflecting on these mortal matters, I find cause for cheer. When I was young and vigorous, mortality fastened me in its hard grip, and the perils of old age are increasingly vivid to me after heart surgery, but as pain and frailty increase through the years, I am less anxious and wrathful. Perhaps a little suffering gives me the authority to speak of scars of various kinds and may give weight to the hope I cherish.

    Dr. Johnson wrote that "every man thinks meanly of himself for not having been a soldier, or not having been at sea." For much of my life I regretted not having been a soldier. I spent two years as an undergraduate in the Army ROTC program, and in my junior year I tried to sign up for the PLC program in the Marine Corps, but my first two years in college were a protracted academic disaster, and my grades were not good enough for the Marines. In 1963 the draft board ordered me to have a physical examination, but I was not drafted, and by 1967 I had had the surgeries that made service impossible. Military service appealed to me because it promised adventure to my naive mind. But, because I took it seriously, it also promised trial by fire and the brotherhood of men at arms. Despite the horrors of war, my friends who are combat veterans are among the sanest people I know. I have learned to make do with other trials. In sickness, as I have experienced it so far, I have had a trial by fire, and the end is not yet. I am a combat veteran of sorts though I have never heard the rattle of guns fired in anger. I claim my father and Jim Kilgo as my companions in arms in the strange battle in which mortification and surrender become the way to victory.

8. EPILOGUE

In the Heaven of Mars in the *Divine Comedy* Cacciaguida tells Dante that his great-grandfather has circled the first ledge of Mount Purgatory for more than a century, and he urges the poet "to shorten his long toil with your good works." Isolated by the horrific events of his childhood, my father closed doors early in his life that he would never reopen. My own trials, starting when I was twenty-five, not eight, have surrounded me with abiding love, and that love also connects the living and the dead and makes sense for me of suffering and pain. The world takes it for madness, but saints have looked upon their sufferings as a gift, an opportunity to participate in the passion of human redemption. And I have begun to think that perhaps my suffering, transformed by the love it has evoked and the desire I have to offer it up, has helped to redeem my father's lonely way even years after his death. The passage of time is no barrier to grace, and the present can illumine the dark corners not only of our own lives but all of the lives that ours can touch back down the years. I have no desire to present myself as the central character in a family saga or to claim sanctity. My task, like Dante's, is simply to recognize my responsibility among the living, my obligation to the dead. I am trying to understand and describe, without exaggeration, the pattern of redemption in life that continues to unfold.

Donald Davidson's poem "Soldier and Son" speaks of the long silence between father and son in which important matters have been left unspoken. The son says that only through conversation can he know his father and asks:

> Without recollection, how can I truly be
> Your son, or a true father of sons?
> What is kindred blood, and no memory?

My father was never able to talk about the things that mattered most in his life: Powell's death and his own and his parents' reaction to it. Unable to speak of those things, he avoided talking about anything deeply personal. In writing about my father, I have tried, more than twenty years after his death, to let him speak. I have tried to be minutely accurate when quoting him, but at this distance I have also seen the drift and pattern of our words, and here on the page we have had the conversation we could not have while he was alive. This is neither woolgathering nor wishful thinking. I believe that human ties are not broken by death. Increasingly in my recollections, I meet the living and the dead on equal terms and find in that both comfort and clarity. There I can hear my father's voice and have the conversation that makes recognition possible.